ASTHMA

OPTIMA

ANSWERS TO
ASTHMA

DR CHRIS SINCLAIR

ILLUSTRATED BY ANDRE YANIW

An OPTIMA book

First published in 1987 by
Macdonald Optima, a division of
Macdonald & Co. (Publishers) Ltd

A BPCC PLC company

BRITISH LIBRARY CATALOGUING IN PUBLICATION DATA

Sinclair, Christopher
    Asthma.—(Healthlines).
    1. Asthma—Treatment
    I. Title   II. Series
    616.2'3806   RC591

    ISBN 0-356-12435-5

Macdonald & Co. (Publishers) Ltd
3rd Floor
Greater London House
Hampstead Road
London NW1 7QX

Photoset in 11/13pt Century by
⊼ Tek Art Limited, Croydon, Surrey

Printed and bound in Great Britain by
The Guernsey Press Company Ltd,
Guernsey,
Channel Islands

CONTENTS

WARNING

Asthma is a serious disease that can be fatal: over 2000 patients die every year in the UK alone. Any asthmatic who is worried about his or her condition should call a doctor or get to a hospital as fast as they can. Early treatment saves lives.

1.
WHAT IS ASTHMA?

Asthma has been recognized since the beginning of medicine as we know it. The word itself is Greek (it means 'panting'), and was first used by the 'father of medicine', the Greek physician Hippocrates, over 2000 years ago. But despite doctors' ability to identify the disease when they see it, they have always remained unable to define it.

Paradoxically, part of the difficulty in defining asthma stems from some of its most characteristic features. First and foremost, asthma is an intermittent disease: even in the most severely affected patients, it is not present all the time – although at times it may seem as though it is. Secondly, although it affects all age groups – with the possible exception of the very young – it tends to affect different age groups in different ways.

Even more confusing for those who try to define asthma is the possibility that other diseases can cause asthma's chief symptom – wheezing. But despite all the difficulties, it is possible to make at least a working definition of asthma. This is important, since it helps doctors to identify those patients who are truly asthmatic, and so are likely to respond to treatment.

Although wheezing is indeed the hallmark of asthma, it is only in fact a symptom – a manifestation – of the underlying disease. The essential factor, which causes the wheezing, is a narrowing of the smaller airways – the bronchi and bronchioles – of the lungs, a process doctors call bronchoconstriction. Furthermore, in the case of asthma, this narrowing is not constant or permanent:

it is 'episodic', varying either spontaneously or as a result of treatment. Taking these two factors into account, doctors define asthma as 'a condition characterized by transient narrowing of the small airways, which (usually) manifests itself in the patient in episodic bouts of wheezy breathing'.

This is, in fact, a very broad definition of asthma. It includes not just one group of patients with asthma, but several, all of which have different characteristics. Overall, however, three main groups can be picked out.

The first group is also the youngest group, and contains those children who develop what are called 'acute wheezy chests'. This condition is most common in children aged between 4 and 8 years old, and tends to disappear by the time they are in their teens.

The next group are the true asthmatics. These individuals may develop their asthma at any age; likewise, it may remain, or disappear, at any time.

The third and last group comprise older patients with chronic bronchitis who develop acute wheezy episodes from time to time. A stricter definition of asthma would not include these patients, but we shall mention them here, since they share many features in common with true asthmatics.

Not surprisingly, such a wide definition of asthma includes many people. Up to 10 per cent of all people may have at least one wheezy episode in their life, but despite this large number, only 2 per cent of the population will be true asthmatics who suffer regularly from the disease.

THE LUNGS AND HOW THEY WORK

It is much easier to understand asthma, what causes it, and how it is treated if we know something of the design of the lungs and how they work.

Our lungs do many things, but their main function is to draw oxygen from the air into our bloodstream, and discharge the waste carbon dioxide from our bodies back into the air. Asthma, as a lung disease, interferes with this process, and not surprisingly the serious effects of asthma are due to the body's lack of oxygen (and, to a lesser extent, an excess of carbon dioxide).

The actual transfer of oxygen from the air to the blood occurs at the end of a long series of tubes, passages and cavities, known collectively as the 'airways' (in much the same way as our digestive system can be described as the 'gut').

Our airways start, of course, at our nose and mouth (see diagram on page 12). Normally we breathe in through the nose, which serves as a combined air filter and conditioner: the air leaving the back of our nose is cleaner, warmer and moister than that entering through our nostrils. Mouths cannot process air in the same way, which is why it is better to breathe through the nose.

Once through the nose, the air enters the combined food and air passage known as the pharynx (throat). At its lower end, the pharynx leads into two separate tubes: the trachea (windpipe) and the oesophagus (food pipe). Food is prevented from going down the trachea by a flap called the epiglottis, or, in an emergency, by the larynx (voice box), which more normally provides the means by which we talk. No mechanism exists, however, to prevent air entering the gut, as we all know to our embarrassment if we eat our food too fast.

Once through the larynx and inside the trachea, the air has entered the specialized air-conducting passageways. These are finely adapted to their job. The lining of the trachea continues the cleaning process started in the nose by means of its sticky mucus covering, to which dirt and germs become attached. Minute hairs, called cilia, sweep the contaminated mucus upwards, and away from the lungs, so that we can either cough the dirt out or swallow it.

The trachea, like an upside-down tree trunk, branches into two main bronchi, one passing to the left lung, the other to the right lung. The bronchi enter the lung, and

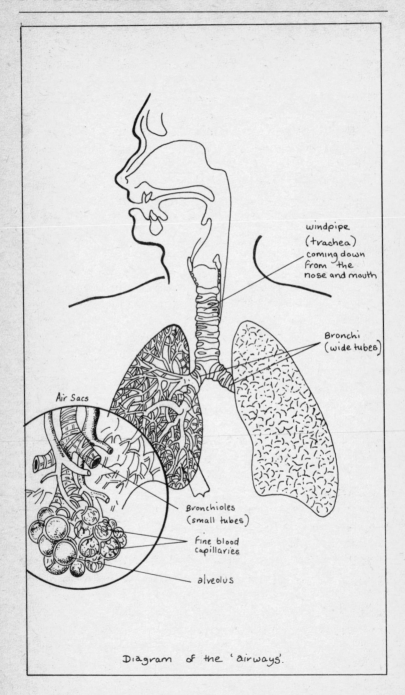

windpipe
(trachea)
coming down
from the
nose and mouth

Bronchi
(wide tubes)

Air Sacs

Bronchioles
(small tubes)

Fine blood
capillaries

alveolus

Diagram of the 'airways'.

divide (like the branches of a tree) into smaller and smaller bronchi. Below a certain size, the bronchi are renamed bronchioles: these are usually about 1mm in diameter.

The last bronchioles, known as the respiratory bronchioles, lead into minute tubes called alveolar ducts, which end in the microscopic sacs, known as alveoli, where the main transfer of gases between the air and the blood occurs.

The 300 million or so alveoli provide a surface area as large as a tennis court, and across this huge surface the gases are exchanged. Immediately alongside the alveoli are the fine blood capillaries, carrying venous, de-oxygenated blood from the right side of the heart. Oxygen diffuses across from the oxygen-rich air to the blood, recharging it, while carbon dioxide is transferred from the blood to the air in the lungs, so that it can be exhaled.

Many lung diseases cause their ill effects by interfering directly with this vital process of gas exchange. Asthma, however, interferes at a different level, and to understand the disease, we need to consider how we get air in and out of our lungs in the process known to doctors as ventilation.

In many respects, the lungs work like a pair of bellows which have been modified by having an elastic band looped round the handles. In the lungs, a series of muscles contract, and in so doing cause the chest to expand. Air is drawn into the lungs and then, as the muscles relax, the chest recoils to its original size, and the air is blown out again.

This process normally goes on, in and out, without our being aware of it, under the control of a special centre in the brain. When we exercise, or become emotionally excited, or something else happens that increases our oxygen requirement, this respiratory centre, as it is called, increases the rate and depth of breathing to meet our body's extra oxygen needs. In the normal, non-asthmatic person, all the airways are of a large enough diameter, and the air flows freely in and out.

WHAT CAUSES ASTHMA?

Now we understand how the lungs work normally, we can appreciate the derangements that occur to cause asthma. Knowing something about the mechanism of asthma, or its 'pathophysiology', as doctors call it, is vital to an understanding of how orthodox medical treatment works, and possibly some of the alternative therapies too.

If we return to our definition of asthma (see page 10), we see that the fundamental process in asthma is a narrowing of the airways. It is this narrowing, rather like pursing the lips when whistling, which causes the audible wheeze. But what is it that causes the airways to become narrower than they should be?

Inside the lungs, there is a network of muscles that spiral round all but the very smallest airways. In the normal person, the function of these muscles is not known, but in the asthmatic they take on a sinister significance. It is the contraction of these muscles (combined, as we shall see, with inflammation and excess phlegm production) which causes the obstruction to the airways that accounts for the asthmatic's misery (see diagram on page 15). These bronchial muscles are of the type known as smooth, or involuntary, muscle – we do not have the same voluntary control over them as we do over for example the muscles in our arms or legs.

The contraction of the bronchial muscle is the cardinal event in asthma, but it does not occur in isolation. Whatever it is that triggers the contraction of the smooth muscle also sets up other reactions in the lung's airways. This reaction is in fact a general type of response of the body to any sort of attack or irritation, and is called inflammation.

Normally, inflammation is a great help, as it enables the body to deal with all sorts of problems, from infections to broken bones and cancer. In asthma, however, it is something of a two-edged sword.

One of the results of inflammation is to cause swelling.

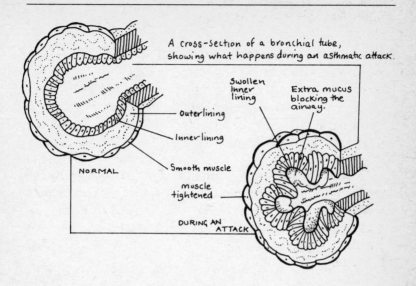

A cross-section of a bronchial tube, showing what happens during an asthmatic attack.

Swollen Inner lining

Extra mucus blocking the airway.

Outer lining

Inner lining

Smooth muscle

muscle tightened

NORMAL

DURING AN ATTACK

This comes about mainly as a result of the collection of fluid, and is known as oedema. Usually the swelling does not cause any great problems, but in the narrow airways of the lungs it is a different matter altogether.

In a person suffering from asthma, the bronchi and bronchioles are already being constricted by the contraction of the smooth muscle. The swelling of the walls of the airways only makes matters worse, reducing yet further the opening through which the air can flow.

Even this is not the end of the story: two more factors combine to make matters even more difficult for the asthmatic. The inflammatory reaction that sets in also causes the lungs to produce more than the usual amount of the thick sticky substance called mucus, or phlegm. This lodges in the narrowed airways, blocking them still further.

Lastly, the actual asthmatic attack itself only makes matters worse. As the asthmatic struggles to breathe out (why the main problem occurs with breathing out will be explained in a moment), air pressure builds up in the chest, pressing on the airways and narrowing them still further. By this stage, a vicious circle has set in.

Asthmatics and people close to them often notice that the main problem in asthma is not so much with breathing in (inhalation), but with breathing out (exhalation). The asthmatic can manage to take a breath in; the difficulty is getting it out again, and it is with the breathing out that the wheeze is produced.

The reason for this seemingly paradoxical situation is tied up with the way in which we breathe. As we breathe in, the pressure in our chest actually goes down, creating a vacuum (that's why the air goes in). This decrease in pressure helps to keep the airways open, by pulling on their walls.

On the other hand, when we breathe out, the pressure goes up, and acts on the walls of the bronchi and bronchioles, so tending to flatten them. This makes them narrower, so making it more difficult to breathe out. This is why the asthmatic experiences the greatest difficult with exhalation, and why the wheeze happens during breathing out.

DIFFERENT KINDS OF ASTHMA

As we saw earlier, on page 10, many different types of people can develop wheezing, although three main groups – children with acute wheezy chests, true asthmatics, and chronic bronchitics who suffer wheezy episodes – can be recognized. Not surprisingly, the disease runs a different course in these different groups. Let us first concentrate on those people who develop true asthma.

Up to 10 per cent of the population may, for one reason or another, be predisposed to develop asthma, but of these, only about one third (i.e. 3-4 per cent of the population) will actually develop the disease proper. Of those who do get true asthma, half will show symptoms before the age of ten, and another third before the age of 40. It is rare for true asthma to appear for the first time after middle age.

If one looks more closely at those people with true asthma, it soon becomes apparent that even in this group

there are different kinds of asthma. Typically, those
patients who develop asthma in childhood tend to have
a different kind of asthma from those who first start to
suffer with the disease later on in life.

Atopic asthma

Individuals who are first diagnosed as having asthma
in childhood tend to have what is known as atopic,
allergic, or extrinsic asthma. Atopy is a subtle concept,
which even today is not fully understood, but it is used
to describe individuals who have certain characteristics,
and who have a tendency to develop a number of allergic
diseases, one of which is asthma.

Atopy is an inherited trait, which, when present, means
that an individual is likely to be more than usually
sensitive to allergens – substances that can provoke an
allergic response. We will look at the allergic response
in greater detail in Chapter 4, but at the moment it is
sufficient to know that atopic people are prone to suffer
from allergic diseases, such as eczema, hay fever – and
asthma.

Because atopy is inherited, atopic asthma tends to run
in families. Even if a relative has not had asthma, there
is often a family history of another atopic disease, such
as eczema. Children born to parents who are both atopic
have a 50 per cent risk of being atopic themselves.

Atopy varies a great deal: some individuals are very
prone to develop multiple allergies; others develop few
or none. Atopy never disappears completely, but it often
improves with age.

Atopic asthmatics have a number of features which
differentiate them from non-atopic asthmatics. One of
the most important is that their attacks of asthma are
often precipitated by identifiable allergens, such as house
dust or pollens. Because atopy is worst in childhood and
improves with age, the asthma, too, tends to start in
childhood, and is often at its most severe then. In many
patients it improves with age, and often disappears with
the onset of puberty.

Atopic, allergic asthma is also known as extrinsic asthma, because as we saw on page 17, the attacks are usually provoked by external allergens. The disease, as well as having a tendency to improve with time, is usually what doctors call episodic – acute attacks occur, with symptom-free intervals in between.

Non-atopic asthma
The other type of true asthma is called non-atopic or intrinsic asthma (and sometimes non-allergic asthma). It is the kind of asthma which tends to appear after childhood, and it differs from atopic asthma in a number of important ways.

Individuals with intrinsic asthma do not have identifiable specific allergens that bring on attacks (although certain other factors can trigger attacks, the mechanism is not allergic). Attacks, when they come, tend to be longer-lasting, and often more serious, and not infrequently the disease becomes chronic (long-lasting), requiring continuous treatment with potent drugs.

Sometimes patients with intrinsic asthma are abnormally sensitive to aspirin and other similar drugs, but as this sensitivity is not a true allergy (it is not brought about through the immune system), it is called aspirin intolerance. Not all patients with aspirin intolerance have asthma, however, and not all patients with intrinsic asthma have aspirin intolerance.

Non-asthmatic acute wheezy chests
These, then are the two types of true asthma. Acute wheezy chests in children, although quite common, are usually less serious than asthma proper. The wheezing often occurs when the child has a cold or a chest infection, and not at other times, and the tendency to wheeze has a habit of disappearing as the child gets older.

Acute wheezy attacks in chronic bronchitis are really a different problem altogether. Chronic bronchitis, as its name suggests, is a long-standing disease, which tends to occur in older people who have smoked for much of their lives. The hallmark of the disease is recurrent bouts of infected phlegm. One of the consequences of chronic bronchitis is a narrowing of the bronchi, leading to obstruction, which is usually permanent. This feature explains why doctors consider chronic bronchitis under the heading of 'chronic obstructive airways disease', or COAD for short (the other disease that comes under this heading is emphysema).

Sometimes, however, the airways obstruction associated with chronic bronchitis is variable. It may therefore be thought of as being (at least to some extent) reversible. Furthermore, when the obstruction is bad, it is often associated with wheezing, and this, combined with its potential reversibility, means that it fits the broader definitions of asthma. It should be clear from what has been said before, however, that true asthma and COAD are not the same disease, although they may be connected. Exacerbations, as doctors call bouts of worsening chronic bronchitis, are often provoked by chest infections, and the treatment differs in many important ways from that of asthma proper.

HOW AN ASTHMATIC ATTACK HAPPENS

Many theories have been put forward to explain how an asthmatic attack happens, but none has gained universal acceptance yet. Central to most, however, is the concept of bronchial hyper-reactivity. Indeed, so important is this concept that many researchers are beginning to believe that it is the central defect in asthma.

Bronchial hyper-reactivity describes a state in which the bronchi (and bronchioles) are abnormally sensitive to a wide range of potential irritants. Whatever it is that causes the reaction, the increased bronchial reactivity ensures that the smooth muscle in the walls of the airways contract, so bringing on an asthmatic attack.

The control of breathing

One theory that has been put forward to explain hyper-reactivity involves the part of the nervous system that controls our breathing, as well as other functions that we are not usually conscious of. This part of the nervous system is called the autonomic nervous system, and it is divided into two sections: the sympathetic and the parasympathetic nervous systems.

The role of the sympathetic nervous system

In health, one of the main jobs of the sympathetic nervous system is to help us respond to threats and stresses by means of the so-called 'flight or fight' response. Among other things, stimulation of the sympathetic nervous system is thought to cause widening of the airways via circulating chemical 'messengers', or hormones, such as adrenaline. This makes breathing easier, and allows the increased requirement of air (including oxygen) to enter the lungs more freely.

It has been suggested that, in asthma, the airways are partially insensitive to the instructions coming from the sympathetic nervous system to widen. Thus they tend to be more constricted than they should be.

Recent research, however, has led doctors to question this traditional view of the role of the sympathetic nervous system. Some of them now believe that either the parasympathetic nervous system or even a different system altogether controls the diameter of the airways. What is certain is that we don't fully understand yet the mechanisms that control the diameter of our airways, and a lot more research still remains to be done.

The actual trigger that causes the narrowing is thought to depend on the kind of asthma the patient has. Attacks in allergic, extrinsic asthma are believed to be caused by extrinsic allergens that act through the immune system. Intrinsic asthma attacks, on the other hand, tend to be triggered by non-specific factors, and it is thought that these may act through the parasympathetic half of the autonomic nervous system as outlined above.

THE EFFECTS OF ASTHMA

Whatever the pathway through which an asthmatic attack is caused, the consequences of the attack are the same. The airways narrow and breathing becomes more difficult than it should be.

On one level, this leads to the asthmatic's symptoms. The sufferer feels short of breath, and finds it especially difficult to breathe out. Wheezing starts, and if the attack becomes more serious, the asthmatic tries to help their lungs to obtain more air by using extra muscles that are not normally used in breathing – the so-called accessory muscles of respiration.

Hyperinflation
Meanwhile, because of the difficulty of breathing out, the air in the lungs becomes trapped there, causing the minute alveolar sacs to blow up like balloons – a process known as hyperinflation. Breathing becomes so difficult that the asthmatic is unable to talk, and, if the attack is especially severe, the actual function of the lungs themselves is interfered with, and the victim starts to go blue, indicating that not enough oxygen is reaching the blood.

MEASURING THE EFFECTS OF ASTHMA

Peak flow meters
As well as producing the dramatic symptoms described above, the effects of asthma show up on a number of tests. First and foremost, asthma affects the speed with which a person can breathe out, and not surprisingly one of the commonest tests used by doctors measures the fastest speed at which the patient can breath air out of the lungs. This is measured by a machine called a peak flow meter into which the asthmatic blows as hard and as fast as they can. The reading is known as the peak expiratory flow rate, or PEFR for short, and is a measure of the

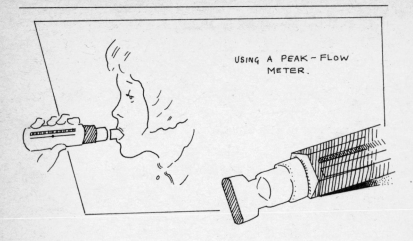

USING A PEAK-FLOW METER.

fastest speed at which the air leaves the lungs. It is expressed in litres per minute.

Although the absolute reading has some importance, the doctor is more interested in the reading as a percentage of what it should be for the individual's age and build. A PEFR considerably lower than expected is highly suggestive of asthma. Even more significant is a reversal of the degree or obstruction following treatment: a 20 per cent or more rise in the PEFR makes it virtually certain that the patient has asthma.

Spirograph tests

Sometimes, more complicated tests are done to assess in greater detail how the asthmatic's lungs are working. Instead of blowing into a peak flow meter, a full breath is exhaled into a different machine called a spirograph. This produces a tracing of the way in which the individual is breathing out, and can give valuable clues about how the lungs are working. Usually, it is clear from the tracing that an asthmatic patient is breathing out more slowly than a normal person.

Other tests

Other 'invisible' abnormalities occur during an asthmatic attack which can, nonetheless, be picked up by laboratory tests. As an attack worsens, the function of the lungs themselves is disturbed. Initially, less oxygen enters the blood, and the asthmatic becomes hypoxaemic ('hypo' means less; 'ox' means oxygen and 'aemic' refers to the blood). Paradoxically, in the early stages, the amount of carbon dioxide in the blood actually falls, but as an attack worsens it soon starts to creep up. Doctors monitor these changes in the blood during serious attacks.

ACUTE SEVERE ASTHMA

Normally, either spontaneously or as a result of treatment, an asthmatic attack is brought under control. Occasionally this does not happen, and for reasons that are not altogether clear, the attack persists and actually worsens, often despite initial treatment. This dangerous situation is known as 'status asthmaticus', or 'acute severe asthma', and it requires attention in hospital (see also pages 33 to 37).

HOW DOES A DOCTOR DIAGNOSE ASTHMA?

Diagnosis of an acute attack of asthma is usually easy, especially in a young person (see pages 104 to 105). It becomes more difficult when the suspected asthmatic is not actually wheezing when seen by the doctor, and in this situation the physician has to look more closely for other clues.

Questions the doctor will ask

The doctor's first step in assessing a person who may have asthma will be to ask them some questions. Some of these questions will be specific, about the breathing problems. Other questions will be more general, and may seem less relevant, but they give the doctor important background information, and sometimes help with the diagnosis of asthma.

The doctor will want to know how old the person is (because different kinds of asthma are more common at different ages), when the attacks start, and whether anything provokes them. The doctor will also want to know what happened during the attack, and how it ended. Recognizing that the attacks are paroxysmal – that is that they come and go – is of paramount importance, for it confirms that the obstruction of the airways is reversible, a hallmark of asthma. The doctor will ask about the patient's own medical history (for example, is there anything to suggest that they are atopic individuals?) and about their family's medical history.

The doctor also needs to assess the severity of the disease, and how it is interfering with the patient's life – for example, how many school or work days are being lost.

Often the answers to the questions will suggest strongly that the patient has asthma, but at other times they will be less conclusive. Whatever the result, the doctor will then examine the possible asthmatic to see if there are any extra clues. If the person is between attacks, there are not likely to be many, although there may be some pointers if the disease is long standing.

Basic tests
The next part of the assessment consists of the special tests that the doctor will do, or arrange to have done. Firstly the peak flow is measured. There follows a chest x-ray, to rule out other lung problems and heart disease, and then examination of the sputum (mucus produced by coughing) to see if it is infected (asthma, as we saw earlier, on page 18, can be triggered by infection).

Sometimes it is still not absolutely clear whether the problem is asthma or not. In this situation, further, more sophisticated tests are needed.

More sophisticated tests
The vitalograph often provides strong evidence of asthma, by showing a reduction in the volume of air that can be forcefully exhaled in one second. Confirmation that the

patient is suffering from asthma can be obtained by giving them a drug that is used to treat asthma, which should have the effect of widening the airways, leading to an improvement in the vitalograph tracing. If this happens, it is virtually certain that the patient is asthmatic.

A doctor may also use other sophisticated tests to help in the diagnosis of asthma. In cases of suspected allergic asthma, allergen testing can be helpful in identifying specific substances which the patient should avoid (see also pages 86 to 89). Exercise tests, in which exercise is used to provoke an attack can provide useful information. Of course, this is done in a safe place, where immediate treatment is available, should the need arise.

Most blood tests in asthmatic patients give normal results. In allergic asthma however, numbers of a particular type of white cell in the blood, called eosinophils, may increase. Eosinophils are cells connected with the allergic response, which is considered in greater detail in Chapter 4, on pages 79 to 86. Chemicals in the blood called antibodies (or immunoglobulins), which are also involved in the allergic response, may show abnormally raised levels on testing.

The only other blood result which may be abnormal in asthma – and then only during particularly bad attacks – is a test known as 'arterial blood gases'. In this test, blood from an artery, rather than venous blood, is used, and it is analysed to see how much oxygen and carbon dioxide it contains. These values become abnormal in severe attacks.

Not all these tests will be carried out on every patient. On many occasions the doctor sees the patient during an attack, and the likelihood of asthma is obvious. Once reversibility of the obstruction to breathing has been demonstrated, the diagnosis is almost certainly asthma, in one of its forms. Even so, many doctors will do some or occasionally all of the tests described above, to improve their understanding of the patient's disease. This extra information can help them to look after the patient in the best possible way.

WHEN IS WHEEZING NOT ASTHMA?

Just as all Australians are human beings, but not all
human beings are Australians, so not all wheezers are
asthmatics. We have already considered the 'semi-
asthmatic' conditions – acute wheezy chests in children,
and temporary bouts of wheezing in chronic bronchitis.
What other diseases can cause confusion with asthma?

In fact, if one excludes the semi-asthmatic diseases,
there is only one condition that is likely to cause
confusion, and this is a particular type of heart failure,
known as left ventricular failure. This condition occurs
when the left side of the heart – the side which pumps
blood around the body – fails, and fluid builds up in the
lungs, as a result of back pressure. This causes, among
other things, wheezing, but other features which
accompany the wheezing in left ventricular failure
usually give the game away. Doctors can usually be
certain what they are dealing with, even in an
emergency.

HOW ASTHMA VARIES WITH TIME

We have already seen how asthma varies over the years.
Young children with extrinsic, allergic asthma
fortunately tend to get better as the years go by. Up to
half of children with mild asthma grow out of their disease
by their teens, but this figure drops to one in five if the
asthma is severe. In a small percentage, asthma can
actually worsen during the teens. Asthma that comes
on in middle age, on the other hand, tends to be more
chronic, and severe attacks are more likely.

The other striking thing about asthma and time is the
remarkable daily variation that occurs in the PEFR (peak
expiratory flow rate – see 'Peak flow meters' on page 21).
In fact, the variations that can occur naturally during
at 24-hour period can exceed the changes due to
treatment, a fact which can be important in assessing
therapy. PEFR readings should, for example, be taken
at the same time of day.

The pattern of change in the PEFR during the day is fairly constant. Generally, it is lowest in the early morning, and highest in the evening. So far, the cause of this variation has not been discovered, but it does explain why some patients experience symptoms mainly at night.

RECENT DEVELOPMENTS IN THE UNDERSTANDING OF ASTHMA

So far, in this chapter, I have described the 'traditional' view of asthma. Recently a number of asthma specialists have begun to question the relative importance of different aspects of asthma.

In particular, some researchers are beginning to doubt whether bronchial smooth muscle contraction is the key event: instead they are beginning to suspect that inflammation is the central event, which leads in turn to the other features, including the smooth muscle spasm.

If this is indeed the case (it is by no means proven yet), it may open the way for a completely new set of drugs for treating asthma. Even if it doesn't achieve this, it will still alter the use of the drugs we already have.

As our understanding of the basic processes that cause asthma has increased, there has been a move to rename asthma – as 'reversible obstructive airways disease', or 'ROAD' for short. Unfortunately, the full name is something of a mouthful, and the shortened version hasn't yet caught on!

2.
ORTHODOX TREATMENT

Not so long ago – certainly in living memory – treatment of asthma was a haphazard business. Doctors did not really understand the nature of the disease, and, not surprisingly, many treatments were not always in the best interests of the patient. In fact, in the light of what we know, some of the treatments that were used were positively dangerous!

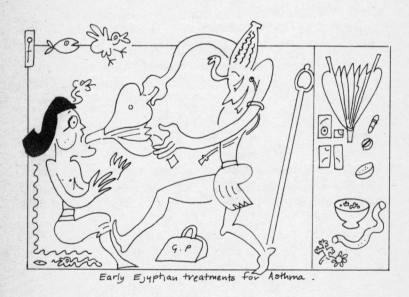

Early Egyptian treatments for Asthma.

The last few decades, however, have seen a dramatic increase in our understanding of the details of asthma, and hand in hand with this increased knowledge has come better, more rational, treatment. Many asthmatics can, with such treatment, lead symptom-free lives. Even so, asthma is still a potentially serious disease that can prove fatal. For this reason alone, the greatest care is always necessary, all the more so because most fatalities seem to occur not so much because the treatment was not available as because no-one realized how serious the situation had become. I shall return to this problem later.

Modern routine treatment of asthma is firmly based on the scientific principles. On pages 10 to 13, I considered how the lungs, and in particular the airways, are made up, and how they work. Given the knowledge we have of the lungs in health and in asthma, it is possible to devise logical therapies that are likely to work.

If we recall (see page 14) that the final process involved in any asthmatic attack is the narrowing of the airways, it is likely that any drug which can prevent or even reverse this process will be effective in asthma. Drugs which cause widening of the airways (bronchodilation) are known as bronchodilators, and are some of the most important ones used to treat asthma.

THE ACUTE ATTACK

Let us look first at how an acute attack of asthma is treated. Narrowing of the airways – bronchoconstriction – is the main problem. As I described earlier (page 20), our autonomic nervous system is important in the control of our airways.

As mentioned already (page 20), one of the chemicals used by the sympathetic nervous system is adrenaline, one of the hormones our body produces when we are under threat. It is adrenaline which makes our mouth go dry and our heart beat faster when we are aware of some danger. In addition (but less obviously to most of us) it dilates the airways, so that we can breathe more easily should the need arise.

ADRENERGIC DRUGS

Adrenaline also gives its name to a whole group of drugs that cause effects similar to the release of adrenaline in the body: they are called adrenergic drugs. Research has shown that there are different classes of adrenergic drugs, depending on which part of the body they actually stimulate.

Adrenergic drugs have therefore been sub-divided into different groups. One group is known as alpha adrenergic agonists (an agonist is a drug that causes the same effects as the substance it is an agonist of), while others are known as beta adrenergic agonists. This latter group has now been divided into two sub-groups – beta-1 and beta-2 agonists. It is the beta-2 agonists that we are interested in, because they are the ones that cause bronchodilation in the lungs.

Adrenaline: powerful but risky

Of the naturally occurring adrenergic drugs, adrenaline is a potent beta-2 agonist, and not surprisingly it is a powerful bronchodilator. Unfortunately, however, its effects are not confined to the lungs (it also has alpha effects), and serious side-effects can develop. For these reasons, it is rarely, if ever, used these days to treat asthma in the UK.

Isoprenaline: a tragic failure

More specific drugs, which would cause marked bronchodilation, but little in the way of side-effects, were needed. One of the earliest contenders was isoprenaline. This drug, however, was still too generalized in effect, and was unfortunately given in high, uncontrolled doses. In the mid-1960s there was a tragic epidemic of sudden deaths in young asthmatics, mainly due to the fact that excessive doses of a powerful drug were being used.

Much of the problem with isoprenaline was that it had both beta-2 and beta-1 effects. The former were of course desirable, and were why the drug worked in treating asthma. The beta-1 effects, which were mainly on the heart, were at best a nuisance, and at worst lethal.

Salbutamol: the life-saver

What was needed was a drug which acted exclusively – or at least mainly – on the beta-2 receptors. The first such drug to be developed was called salbutamol. Today, this drug is still the mainstay of asthmatic treatment, and it probably true to say that more asthmatics owe their lives to this drug than to any other development in the treatment of asthma.

The advantages of salbutamol

Salbutamol has a number of distinct advantages in the treatment of asthma. First and foremost, it is tailor-made for its purpose: as a beta-2 adrenergic agonist (with only slight beta-1 effects) it is capable of achieving the bronchodilation that is required, without causing a threat to the asthmatic's life through its action on the heart.

Secondly, it can be administered to an asthmatic in a number of ways, including by inhaler. This is highly significant, since it means that the drug can be got where it is needed straight away. Various systems exist to deliver the drug by inhalation (I will shortly describe the details of these systems) but the important point is that the drug is got to where it is needed.

Let us return now to the asthmatic who is suffering an acute attack. For whatever reason (it doesn't matter what the trigger is at this stage), the smooth muscle in the patient's airways has gone into spasm, and bronchoconstriction has resulted. What is needed is something to bring about relaxation of the muscle, so that the airways can dilate again, thus easing the breathing problems.

This is where salbutamol comes in. Because it is a selective beta-2 agonist, which can be delivered by inhalation, it gets straight to where the problem is – the bronchi – where it can start working immediately.

Not surprisingly, therefore, salbutamol is the mainstay

in the treatment of an asthmatic attack, whether it is in the early stages, and being treated by the patient himself or herself, or whether it has already deteriorated to the point where a doctor is needed.

Salbutamol inhalers

In the early stages, most asthmatics will treat themselves, with a device called an inhaler. This gadget is really an upside-down aerosol, designed to deliver a metered dose of dry salbutamol, which the patient breathes in, using a special technique. So widespread is this device amongst asthmatics that most attacks are controlled in their early stages by the use of salbutamol inhalers.

Nebulizers

Should the salbutamol inhaler not be sufficient to bring the attack under control, there is a second method of inhaling the drug which is often beneficial in this situation. The second system relies on a device called a nebulizer, and it differs from an inhaler in two important ways.

The first and most important difference is that a nebulizer uses a salbutamol *solution*. This means that the 'air' entering the asthmatic's lungs is moist, and therefore less irritant. Secondly, the gas that drives the nebulizer, and makes it work, is usually oxygen, which is also vital to an asthmatic suffering a moderately severe attack. Indeed, asthmatics need and should be given oxygen during a serious attack whether they are using a nebulizer or not.

Nebulizers are not without their disadvantages, though. A supply of gas is necessary to make them work, and for this reason they are not easily used outside hospital. However, it is probably true to say that many attacks which are bad enough to need a nebulizer are also bad enough to need hospital attention.

HOSPITAL TREATMENT

Returning now to our asthmatic patient, let us suppose
that the attack is quite a bad one, and hospital treatment
is indeed necessary. (Sometimes GPs use some of the
methods practised in hospital, but as GPs vary
tremendously in their treatment of an asthmatic attack,
it is easier if I consider here just what happens in
hospital.)

Once in the hospital, the first task is usually an attempt
to measure the patient's peak flow. It often is only an
attempt, without much success, because of the difficulty
of blowing into the meter during a bad attack. But even
if no reading is obtained, the failure still provides helpful
information to the doctors and nurses who are looking
after the patient, as it tells them that they are faced with
a fairly severe attack.

Assessing the seriousness of an attack

Once the peak flow has been recorded, most doctors will
make a quick assessment of how serious the attack is.
This may be difficult, but usually the doctor can rely on
certain pointers, or 'physical signs' as they are called,
to tell him how bad things are.

Some of the signs of a serious attack are more obvious
than others. Inability to talk, because of the difficulty
with breathing, is an obvious sign. So too is the use of
the so-called accessory muscles of respiration – muscles
we don't normally use to breathe with – to try and help
move air in and out of the lungs. Use of these extra
muscles is often associated with a particular posture.

Another obvious sign, this time indicating that the
attack is a very bad one, is if the victim goes blue, an
effect known medically as cyanosis. Cyanosis indicates
that there is far too little oxygen in the blood, which is
an ominous sign.

Other signs may be less immediately obvious, but are
nonetheless very important in assessing the patient. A
high heart rate suggests a serious attack (bearing in mind

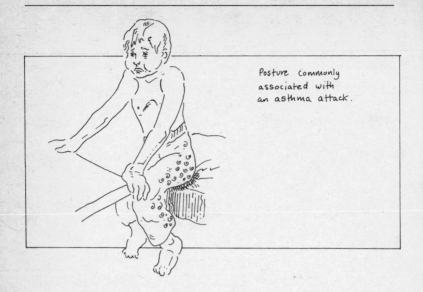

Posture commonly associated with an asthma attack.

that anxiety can also cause the heart to beat faster), as does the development of a characteristic change in the blood pressure, known as pulsus paradoxus (this is what doctors are referring to when they say there is so many millimetres of paradox).

Last, but not least, there is the wheezing. It might be thought that the worse the attack, the worse the wheeze, and up to a point this is true. Beyond this point, however, the airways have become so narrow that hardly any air is getting in or out. This situation is known as a 'silent chest', and is indicative of a very severe and possibly life-threatening attack.

Deciding on the best treatment
Taking all these various signs into account (usually as quickly as possible, so as not to delay treatment any longer than is necessary), the doctor can decide on the best form of treatment.

On many occasions, when the attack is not very severe, a salbutamol nebulizer is the first line of treatment. Often this brings a rapid marked improvement, easing the breathing and allowing the victim to start to talk.

Treating a severe attack

Sometimes, however, the nebulizer is not enough to bring the attack under control on its own. Alternatively, it might have been obvious from the beginning that the attack was a particularly severe one, a condition known as status asthmaticus (status asthmaticus is the medical term for a prolonged asthmatic attack, which has not been brought under control by the patient's usual medication). In these situations, further measures are needed to assess and control the attack.

One of the problems in a severe attack is that the airways are too narrowed to allow any drug that is inhaled to get to where it is needed. In this situation an alternative means of getting the drug to the scene of the problem is needed. The method used is to give the drug by injection into a vein.

The intensely narrowed airways also prevent the patient from blowing into the peak flow meter. An alternative test is needed to assess the severity of the attack, and the one that is used is to measure the amount of oxygen (and carbon dioxide) in the asthmatic's arterial blood. Sooner or later a chest X-ray will also be done.

Up to this point, there is relatively little controversy amongst doctors about what the best course of action is. When the situation is reached where intravenous treatment is needed, however, experts sometimes disagree about the best drug to use.

Until recently, most doctors would have used two drugs: a steroid, and, because a steroid can take up to six hours to work, another drug to act immediately. In the UK, this second drug has usually been aminophylline (see also page 41).

Aminophylline is unfortunately not without its problems. It is a relatively toxic drug, and the difference between a dose large enough to control an attack and an overdose is not that great. This is a great problem in patients who use aminophylline in the routine day-to-day treatment of their asthma, where an extra dose given in the casualty ward of a hospital can put them into the toxic range. For this reason, doctors always check whether a patient is taking aminophylline before proceeding to use it in an emergency.

These problems have encouraged doctors to try and find alternative drugs that can be used to provide immediate relief in severe attacks. Nowadays more and more specialists are recommending the use of intravenous salbutamol, the same drug that is usually given by inhaler or nebulizer. Injecting it into a vein during a bad attack makes sure it gets to where it is needed, as it is carried to the bronchi by the bloodstream. In this way the obstruction in the airways is avoided.

When aminophylline is used, it has to be injected slowly, over about 10 minutes. This time can seem like eternity to an anxious patient – and to the doctor. Salbutamol, on the other hand, can be injected much faster.

Regardless of which bronchodilator is used, a steroid will also be given to help reduce the inflammation in the airways (swelling and inflammation, remember, contribute to the obstruction in severe asthma). Steroid injections are usually continued for a further two days or so, when a switch is made to tablets.

Rare complications
The combined treatment with a bronchodilator and a steroid is almost always sufficient to bring an asthmatic attack under control. Very rarely, the situation continues to get worse. Luckily, this only happens in about 1 per cent of asthmatics with status asthmaticus.

When it does happen, though, it constitutes a grave threat to the patient's life, and definite action is necessary. The asthmatic will be losing consciousness, and death is not far away.

Assisted ventilation
What doctors do in this situation is to help the patient to breathe through a technique known as assisted ventilation. A tube, called an endotracheal tube, is passed

down into the trachea, and a mechanical ventilator pumps a mixture of oxygen and other gases into the patient's lungs, so relieving the exhausted muscles of the work. As the gas is not pumped in continuously, this type of assisted ventilation is known as intermittent positive pressure respiration (IPPR). Clearly, a patient requiring this sort of treatment will be admitted to an intensive therapy unit.

There are of course risks in giving an aggressive treatment like assisted ventilation, but the risks of not using the techniques are even greater.

Until now, we have only considered acute attacks of asthma. Much of the time, of course, asthmatics are not suffering an acute attack. Nevertheless, all but the mildest asthmatics need medication to try and prevent attacks. This treatment is known as maintenance therapy.

MAINTENANCE THERAPY

Many of the drugs used in maintenance therapy are, not surprisingly, the same drugs that are used to treat acute attacks: regularly taking the drug keeps attacks at bay. Again, as with the treatment of acute asthma, there is a series of graded treatment programmes. There are also treatments which are only useful in the prevention of attacks: these are of no use once an attack has started.

The mainstay of maintenance treatment are the beta-2 agonists, especially salbutamol (see pages 31 and 32). Tablets, although they exist, are not usually the best way of giving the drug: instead an inhaler is used, the asthmatic taking one or two metered puffs from a pressurized aerosol inhaler three or four times a day.

Inhalers
Inhalers are a particularly good way to give a drug to an asthmatic. Firstly, some of the drug (not all of it – some gets waylaid, as explained below) gets directly to where it is needed, meaning not only that it starts

working rapidly, but also that a lower dose of the drug can be used. Side effects, which occur when the drug enters the bloodstream, are kept to a minimum.

Interestingly, not all of an inhaled dose passes into the bronchi. In fact, only about 10 per cent reaches the lungs directly: the rest becomes stuck on the walls of the throat and is swallowed. Inhaled therapy should therefore be thought of more correctly as combined inhaled/oral therapy, although of course the important point is that at least some is being inhaled.

Problems of inhalers

Inhalers also have their problems. The most important one is that not everyone finds inhalers easy to use. There is a necessary technique which young children, the elderly and confused, and people with bad arthritis often find difficult to manage. To get the drug to where it is needed, the asthmatic has to co-ordinate firing the inhaler with breathing in. Although it doesn't sound too difficult, it is in fact much easier said than done.

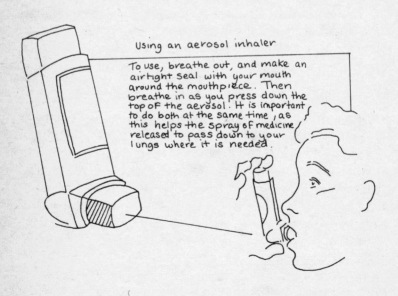

Using an aerosol inhaler

To use, breathe out, and make an airtight seal with your mouth around the mouthpiece. Then breathe in as you press down the top of the aerosol. It is important to do both at the same time, as this helps the spray of medicine released to pass down to your lungs where it is needed.

There are various ways of getting round this problem. Special modifications can be made to the inhaler (in the form of spacing devices) to increase the chances of the drug being inhaled, even if breathing in and firing the inhaler aren't perfectly co-ordinated. Alternatively, instead of having a pressurized aerosol provide the drug, it can be released into a rotocap device (a spinhaler or rotahaler) actually triggered by the patient taking in a breath.

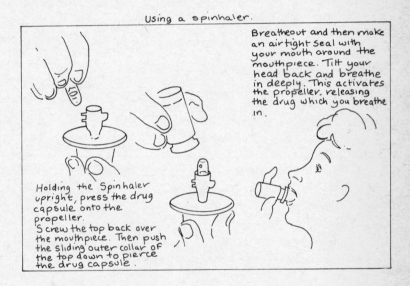

Using a spinhaler.

Breathe out and then make an airtight seal with your mouth around the mouthpiece. Tilt your head back and breathe in deeply. This activates the propeller, releasing the drug which you breathe in.

Holding the Spinhaler upright, press the drug capsule onto the propeller. Screw the top back over the mouthpiece. Then push the sliding outer collar of the top down to pierce the drug capsule.

Sometimes, nebulizers (see page 32) are provided for home use, although this does not happen very often, because of the expense involved, as the equipment is not available for home use on the NHS. As well as being expensive, they are also relatively bulky and unportable. Many patients who use them like them, and say that the bronchodilation achieved is better than that from dry inhalers. Strictly speaking, however, this improved effect has not been demonstrated by laboratory tests. Furthermore, the dose of drug administered via a nebulizer is many times larger than that given through an inhaler, and although this makes the treatment more effective, there is also a slightly increased risk of an overdose.

Tablets

Should inhaled therapy, for whatever reason, not prove suitable, the drug can, of course, be taken by mouth as tablets. Irritating side effects, such as tremor and nevous tension, are more common. Luckily, these side-effects wear off as the drug is taken over a period of time. Dangerous cardiac side effects are virtually unknown with the modern selective beta-2 drugs such as salbutamol.

Alternatives to beta adrenergic drugs

The beta adrenergic agonist drugs are not the only drugs used to treat asthma. Which other drugs (if indeed any) are used depends on a number of factors, including the type and severity of the asthma, and also where the asthmatic lives.

The second main group of drugs, after the beta-agonists, are known as the xanthine derivatives, a group including the well-known social drug caffeine, which provides the 'pick-me-up' effect of coffee. The important ones from an asthmatic's point of view, however, are theophylline and its water-soluble relation, aminophylline (see also page 41).

Theophylline

Theophylline is a potent drug which has a number of effects, including stimulation of the heart. It is also a diuretic – that is, it stimulates urine production. More importantly for asthmatics, it relaxes smooth muscle, both in blood vessels, causing an effect known as vasodilation, and in the bronchi, so causing bronchodilation. Theophylline itself does not dissolve easily in water, which does not affect the production of tablets, but interferes with the making of solutions. For this reason, especially in this country, a modified drug, known as aminophylline, which *is* soluble in water, is commonly used. For this reason, I will refer mainly to aminophylline, as it is the drug most asthmatics are likely to be familiar with.

Aminophylline

Aminophylline is very much a two-edged sword. Unlike the beta agonists, in which there is a great difference between the dose needed to achieve the desired effect and a toxic dose, aminophylline has what is known as a low therapeutic index. This is just the pharmacologists' (scientists who study drugs) technical way of saying that there is not that much difference between a useful dose and an overdose.

Fortunately, there are easy ways to measure the amount of aminophylline in the blood, and so check whether the level is in the safe but effective range. This is especially important, because people vary in the speed at which they break down aminophylline in their bodies, so that what might be the correct dose for one person might constitute an overdose for another. On the other hand, for patients who break the drug down more rapidly, a given dose might be inadequate. All this needs to be taken into account when prescribing the drug.

Many of aminophylline's side effects are predictable from its pharmacological actions. Like theophylline, it is a potent vasodilator, relaxing the smooth muscle in blood vessels, and this can lead to headaches and a lowering of blood pressure. It also stimulates the nervous system, causing tremor and restlessness. Stomach irritation, resulting in nausea and vomiting, also occurs.

With higher levels of aminophylline in the blood, much more serious side-effects can develop, including convulsions and even sudden death from effects on the heart. Generally, these side effects are extremely rare, but the possibility is always lurking in the background, which is why doctors need to be careful in the way they use the xanthine derivative drugs.

Combination therapy

As mentioned earlier, American doctors tend to favour theophylline as a first-line drug in the treatment of even mild asthma. In Europe, the beta-agonists are usually used as the first-line drugs, but sometimes unacceptable amounts of even these drugs are needed. Rather than increase the dose regardless, combination therapy, involving several drugs, is often used, allowing lower doses of the individual drugs. The xanthine derivatives are also useful when inhaled therapy is not suitable, as, for example, in very young patients.

Xanthine derivatives are broken down rather rapidly by the body, so that even with regular, round-the-clock administration, blood levels of the drug fluctuate, increasing the chances of both overdosing and underdosing. This problem has been countered by the development of slow-release preparations which, after being swallowed, release the drug gradually, rather than all in one go. In this way, only two or three doses are needed each day, and there is a further advantage that blood levels remain adequate, even during the night, when some patients are particularly prone to suffer attacks.

Two other groups of drugs that were widely used to treat asthma in the past, but are less important these days, are expectorants and drugs known as anti-cholinergics.

Expectorant drugs

Expectorants (cough-promoting drugs) were used to try and counter the build-up of sticky mucus (phlegm) in the lungs that is known to be part of the problem in an asthmatic attack. Modern research has shown that, at least in this respect, expectorants have little to offer the asthmatic, although they may of course be useful in treating other conditions, such as bronchitis.

Anti-cholinergic drugs

Anti-cholinergics, however, do have an effect. As I

described earlier, on page 20, the airways are controlled, at least to some extent, by the autonomic nervous system. Stimulation by the sympathetic nervous system causes bronchodilation, while stimulation by the parasympathetic nerves causes bronchoconstriction. Anti-cholinergics are drugs that block the effects of the parasympathetic nerves, and, not surprisingly, by blocking nerves that cause constriction, result in widening of the airways (bronchodilation).

In the early days of the treatment of asthma, anti-cholinergic drugs were made up into cigarettes and cigars, which, somewhat ironically, given our modern views on smoking, were effective. Unfortunately (rather like the adrenergic drugs) their effects were more widespread than was needed, because they affected all the parasympathetic nervous system.

Luckily, it is possible to modify some anti-cholinergic drugs so that they are poorly absorbed into the blood. If the drug is then taken in by an inhaler, it acts in the lungs, causing bronchodilation, but does not spread elsewhere. Such a drug is ipratropium. For reasons that are not entirely clear, this drug is far more effective against the reversible element of airways obstruction that can occur in chronic bronchitis than it is against allergic and exercise-induced asthma.

Despite all the drugs I have mentioned so far, some of which are usually very effective, there still remains a group of asthmatics who do not respond adequately to these treatments. They need a still stronger form of therapy, which today is provided by using steroids.

Steroid treatment
As I described earlier (pages 35 to 36), steroids are often used in hospital to treat severe acute attacks of asthma. They are given by injection, or through a drip, and, although high doses are used, this does not usually matter, because the dose is soon reduced as the attack is brought under control.

Using steroids for day-to-day maintenance therapy is

a different matter altogether, however. Not only are they potent drugs, with marked and often unpleasant side effects, but also they cannot be stopped abruptly, once a patient has become used to them.

The term 'steroid' covers a vast range of compounds, but those important in medicine are known as corticosteroids, after the cortex of the adrenal gland, where many of the body's naturally occuring steroids are produced. These natural corticosteroids are hormones and are involved in the control of a wide variety of natural processes. Generally, however, their effects can be divided into two main categories, glucocorticoid and mineralocorticoid, and they are classified according to which category their effects mainly fall into. The group important as asthma drugs are the glucocorticosteroids, which are often known as 'steroids' for short.

The key property of steroids which makes them so useful in the treatment of asthma is their anti-inflammatory effect. Asthma, as we discussed earlier, involves at least three processes, of which one is inflammation (the other two are bronchoconstriction and the build-up of mucus, or phlegm, in the airways). Glucocorticosteroids are potent anti-inflammatory agents, and this is why they are so effective in treating asthma.

Hydrocortisone and prednisolone
The steroid normally used to control an acute attack of asthma is hydrocortisone. This particular steroid unfortunately also has mineralocorticoid effects, and so is unsuitable for long-term therapy, because of the side effects that would develop (short-term use to control a severe attack does not allow enough time for these side effects to develop).

One of the most commonly used steroids for regular treatment of asthma is a synthetic compound known as prednisolone. This particular steroid is a far more potent anti-inflammatory agent than hydrocortisone on a dose-for-dose basis, and furthermore, it has little mineralocorticoid effect.

Even so, most, if not all, cells in our bodies have steroid receptors, so that any steroid which is given by mouth, and so gets into the bloodstream, will have widespread effects. Prednisolone is no exception. These effects become more marked the longer the therapy is continued for, and the higher the dose.

Side effects of steroids

One of the most serious side effects of steroids is, ironically, the very effect for which they are used in the first place – their anti-inflammatory action. This is because of the importance of the inflammatory response in protecting us against many hazards, most notably infection. It is through the process of inflammation that we fight off infections ranging from the common cold to life-threatening pneumonia. Anti-inflammatory drugs weaken our resistance to infections by suppressing the inflammatory response.

As well as causing this problem, steroids unfortunately have a large catalogue of adverse side effects. Clearly, not all asthmatics will suffer from all the side effects that

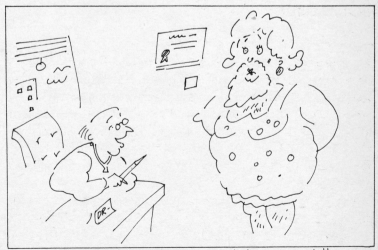

Right Mrs. Smith, the steroids seem to have cleared the asthma up altogether ... Err ... Any other problems?

are described here. Nonetheless, it is wise to be aware that they exist, so as to be alert to the possibility should any of them develop.

One of the most common side effects is weight gain, caused by the deposition of fat in a characteristic manner, mainly around the trunk. The appetite increases, and asthmatics on steroids need to watch their calorific intake. Ironically, at the same time, muscle breakdown increases, causing thinning of the arms and legs. The combination of a fat trunk and thin limbs leads to an appearance that has, somewhat unfairly, been described as looking like a potato with matchstick arms and legs.

The bones can become abnormally weak through a process known as osteoporosis, and in certain cases fractures can result, typically in the vertebrae of the spine. Attention to diet, and possibly vitamin D supplements, can help to reduce the risk of this unpleasant side effect.

Steroids also interfere with the way in which our bodies handle sugar, and in susceptible people this can lead to the development of diabetes mellitus. Hypertension (high blood pressure) may also be worsened.

The skin also undergoes characteristic changes, becoming thin and often bruised, and covered in stretch marks. Acne and increased hairiness (hirsutism) are common in teenagers, and can be a particular embarrassment for girls. Growth, while children are still growing, is inhibited, and children treated continuously with steroids will be shorter than they might have been.

The eyes can be affected, too, leading to glaucoma and cataracts. Mental changes also occur, leading to either depression or some other form of mental illness. Stomach pains are also common, although the belief in the past that steroids caused peptic ulcers is no longer thought to be justified. Steroids can, however, through their anti-inflammatory effects, mask the symptoms of a perforated ulcer, leading to dangerous delay in treatment.

Taking steroids also suppresses our own natural

production of steroids. This is of relatively little importance while the steroid therapy is continuing, but it does mean that abrupt withdrawal of the drug can be dangerous. This hazard is combated by a gradual reduction in the dose of the steroid, rather than suddenly ending the treatment, when the time comes to stop steroid use.

All these side-effects may make it sound as though taking steroids is not worth the risk for asthmatics. Certainly, in mild cases of asthma most doctors believe there is little justification for the use of oral steroids, but as the severity of the asthma increases, so the scales start to weigh more heavily in favour of using steroids. Even when steroids are considered necessary, the dose should be kept to a minimum, and the duration of treatment kept as short as possible. Luckily, such guidelines mean that most asthmatics do not suffer serious side-effects when they are treated with steroids.

Beclomethasone: a new steroid drug
The risks of steroid therapy in asthma were considerably reduced in the 1970s when a new steroid called beclomethasone was first introduced. This drug differs from existing steroids in a number of important ways. Firstly, it could be inhaled, and secondly, very little of the drug ever gets into the bloodstream. In this way, the drug is delivered exactly where it is needed, and unwanted side effects are kept to a minimum.

Levels of beclamethasone are kept low in the bloodstream by a rather ingenious mechanism. The drug from the inhaler is in fact absorbed, but, as we heard earlier, this is because approximately 90 per cent or so of a drug from an inhaler aerosol is actually swallowed. Only a small amount of the drug enters the bloodstream from the lungs. The majority of the drug that has been swallowed is actually absorbed, but only a small amount reaches the rest of the body, as most of the drug is broken down in the liver before it ever reaches the rest of the circulation.

The arrival of beclomethasone solved many of the problems associated with the use of steroids to treat asthma. Even so, steroids are still not often used as first-line drugs in asthma. Nor, unfortunately, is beclomethasone strong enough to control very severe asthma: in this situation steroid tablets are still necessary.

Balancing the benefits and the risks associated with the steroid treatment of asthma is never easy. It is important for the doctor to keep a sense of perspective, and not be unduly hesitant to use steroids when they are genuinely needed. More asthmatics probably die from under-use, rather than over-use, of steroids.

PREVENTING ATTACKS USING SODIUM CROMOGLYCATE

Sodium cromoglycate is a drug that is useful in preventing attacks in allergic (extrinsic) asthma. Unlike most of the other drugs we have considered, it is of no help in treating established attacks, for it works in a totally different way. Allergic asthmatic attacks occur through a complex mechanism (explained in greater detail in Chapter 4, on pages 79 to 86), and sodium cromoglycate acts by blocking one of the steps in this reaction. In this way, although the asthmatic is exposed to the allergen, no attack occurs. Because of the way in which it works, the drug has to be taken by inhaler.

Sodium cromoglycate is also sometimes helpful in preventing exercise-induced asthma. As exercise-induced attacks are not a result of allergy, this suggests that sodium cromoglycate must also act in some other additional way to prevent attacks.

HYPOSENSITIZATION

Some readers may wonder why I have not yet discussed hyposensitization (more correctly but less commonly called immunotherapy). The reason is that it is one of the more controversial areas in the treatment of asthma.

Before reading what follows, some readers may find it helpful to go through the section on allergy in Chapter 4, on pages 79 to 86.

The use of small doses of a substance to prevent the adverse effects of greater exposure, which forms the essence of immunotherapy, may sound more akin to homeopathy than orthodox medicine. In fact, the technique was pioneered by a Dr Noon as long ago as 1911, and so has been around for some considerable time. Despite this, there is still no consensus on whether it is a valid therapy that can be used to prevent asthma.

How immunotherapy may work

Before scientists had unravelled the secrets of immunology (the scientific study of natural immunity to disease), certain diseases, hay fever amongst them, were thought to be due to a toxin, or poison, given off by pollen. Gradually increasing exposure was believed to lower the patient's susceptibility to the poison, but clearly this is not the explanation.

Even today, however, when we have some knowledge of how allergic diseases are caused, we are far from certain how immunotherapy might work. Nonetheless scientists, with their usual ingenuity, have managed to put forward some interesting ideas.

The immunoglobulin theory

The most popular theory involves immunoglobulins (antibodies), but not those of the IgE type (see Chapter 4, page 82) that are so intimately involved in the causation of allergic asthma. According to this theory, injection of dilute quantities of the allergen causes us to produce antibodies to the allergen. This time, however (because the allergen has been injected), different antibodies are formed, mainly of the IgG class (see Chapter 4, page 82). It is suggested that these IgG antibodies get to the allergen and 'mop it up' before it can react with the IgG antibody and provoke an asthmatic attack.

Attractive as this theory sounds, it starts to look less convincing when it is realized that only very small amounts of IgE are released into the airway secretions. It is difficult to understand how the mopping-up of the allergen by IgG antibodies could work when so little IgG reaches the place where it is needed.

Other theories to explain immunotherapy
Other ideas that have been put forward include decreased sensitivity of mast cells and reduced IgE secretion. None of these are proven, and, for the time being at least, it appears that doctors will have to put up not only with being unsure of how the process might work, but of whether it even works at all.

What is involved in immunotherapy treatment?
Putting aside the question of how and whether immunotherapy works, let us consider the way in which the treatment is carried out, as undoubtedly many asthmatics will encounter the technique. Clearly, if it is to be effective, it is essential that true allergens are identified. This requires rigorous skin testing and very careful assessment of the results. There is no point in desensitizing someone to pollen when they are not allergic to it, or for that matter desensitizing a patient to the house dust mite (see page 89) when it plays only a minor role in causing their asthma!

The extracts used in the treatment also have to be of a high and consistent quality. A number of different methods are used for extracting the allergen, but the most common involves the use of water-based solutions. Generally, single component extracts are preferred. One or two known allergens which the doctor is sure that the patient will be exposed to are usually chosen. Seasonal asthma (such as pollen-induced asthma) is easier to treat than asthma that is present all the year round.

The timing of the injections is also important. Levels of IgE, not unexpectedly, actually *rise* during the first stage of the treatment, and take some time to fall (possibly because of the delay while the blocking IgG antibody is being made). For this reason, treatment is best started up to six months before the time of maximum exposure to the allergen, for example, the pollen season.

Injections are given under the skin in the arm. Initial doses are low, and then increasing doses are given until the maximum dose is reached. This is then used as the maintenance dose until the pollen season starts, when the treatment is discontinued until the following year. There is some evidence that repeated courses improve the benefit that is obtained.

Methods of assessing the actual dose that should be given vary from doctor to doctor. Often a standard low initial dose is used, and this is doubled at each injection, providing there have been no untoward general symptoms or exaggerated response at the injection site. The highest dose which can be tolerated without the patient reacting becomes the maintenance dose. Although injections may at first be necessary every few days, usually every three to four weeks is sufficient during the maintenance phase.

Treatment can last as long as the patient benefits, typically for three to five years. No improvement after a year is an indication to stop treatment. Temporary reduction in the dose is usually necessary if the patient has a chest infection or has asthmatic symptoms at the time of the injection. Excessive reactions to the last injection given, as described above, indicate that the subsequent dose should be reduced.

Who benefits most from immunotherapy?
This is how immunotherapy is carried out, but the question still remains as to whether it works. Clearly the prerequisite discussed above – the identification of a known allergen – is essential. In this ideal situation, pollen-induced asthma appears to respond best to immunotherapy, while mite allergy sometimes benefits. In general, the younger the patient, the greater the benefit.

The risks of immunotherapy

Immunotherapy is not without its hazards, as might be predicted from the fact that allergens are being used to treat an allergic disease. There is always the risk that the patient may develop a major, life-threatening allergic response, and in fact at the time of writing there have been at least five deaths in the last 18 months alone from the use of immunotherapy. The doctor who is giving the treatment should always be aware of the possibility, and have the necessary drugs and equipment for treatment to hand, and the patient should always understand that there is a risk involved.

Many specialists in the treatment of asthma make the point that a similar degree of control of symptoms can be more easily achieved by using inhaled therapy, which is safe, simple, and also saves the patient the nuisance and discomfort of repeated injections.

OTHER CONSIDERATIONS IN THE TREATMENT OF ASTHMA

So far I have considered only the direct treatment of both acute and chronic asthma. As so frequently happens in medicine, there are often factors – perhaps those bringing on an acute attack, or even side effects resulting from treatment – that also need attention.

Infection

I have already described direct treatments for a number of causes bringing on an attack earlier in this chapter. One relatively common cause of a worsening in the asthmatic's condition that has not been fully covered is infection. Although different infections tend to be responsible at different ages, there is no doubt that any acute infection can have serious consequences for an asthmatic.

Most chest infections tend to be caused by viruses, as opposed to bacteria. Strange as it may seem, it can actually be a bad thing to treat a viral infection with antibiotics (which are effective only against bacteria), and for this reason, most doctors will avoid antibiotics unless there is good evidence that a bacterial lung infection is part of the problem. Luckily, recognition of bacterial infections is not difficult, and easily proven by laboratory tests. When such an infection is present, antibiotics will be given along with any other treatment that is necessary.

Dehydration

Another difficult area in the treatment of an acute attack of asthma is the dehydrating effect of the attack. Both the breathlessness (making it difficult to drink) and the increased fluid lost in the breath contribute to the drying effect of acute severe asthma. The resulting dehydration itself then causes problems, for example increasing the stickiness and tenacity of the mucus (phlegm), making it more likely to block the airways.

The way doctors treat this dehydration is by giving fluid through a drip. This has the added advantage that drugs can be administered directly into the bloodstream, without the need for repeated injections. Furthermore, potassium levels in the blood frequently drop during treatment of severe asthma (mainly as a side effect of the drugs used), and a drip provides a convenient way of giving supplements of this important mineral in the blood. Abnormally low levels of potassium cause weakness and malaise.

Clearing mucus

After an acute attack of asthma is over, patients frequently cough up much of the sticky mucus, or phlegm, that has been contributing to the airways' obstruction. Normally, most of the mucus comes up of its own accord, but sometimes physiotherapy is needed to help free the more tenacious secretions.

SCIENTIFIC BASIS OF ASTHMA TREATMENT

Throughout this chapter, I have discussed treatments

in a way which has assumed that they work (or clearly said when they did not). This is not, I believe, an unreasonable approach, but certain readers might well ask themselves: how do I know that a particular treatment works – or, for that matter, doesn't work, as is possibly the case for much of immunotherapy. The answer lies in a technique called the randomized controlled clinical trial.

The randomized controlled clinical trial (or RCCT for short) is one of the most important – if not the most important – research development in medicine since the war, for it is the means by which doctors test whether a particular treatment works. It is through the application of RCCTs that doctors have gained the knowledge and the confidence to treat asthma scientifically.

The idea behind RCCTs is extremely simple, even if the subsequent statistical calculations are not. Firstly, to assess a particular treatment, a group of patients who receive the treatment are compared to a group who do

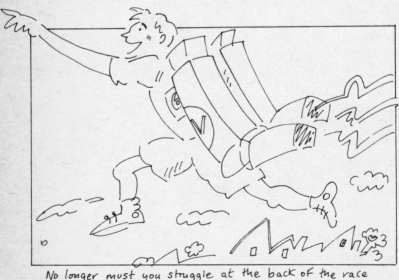

No longer must you struggle at the back of the race
use ⸻ VENTOLIN.

not. This forms what is called a *clinical trial*.

Because, however, unforeseen differences between the groups, or their treatments, could influence the result, rigorous control of all factors that could affect the result (except of course the treatment itself!) is necessary: hence the term *controlled* clinical trial. Finally, to make doubly sure that bias doesn't creep in, patients are allocated at random to either the treatment or the non-treatment group. This makes the trial *randomized*, and so gives it its full, rather long-winded title.

Properly conducted, RCCTs are capable of showing beyond any reasonable doubt that either a treatment works or it doesn't. Unfortunately, not all RCCTs are carefully designed and flawlessly carried out. Nonetheless, good trials have been done, and doctors now know that certain treatments work.

Herein lies the crux of the matter. Asthma is always a serious disease: even today, it claims far more lives every year than it should do (why these tragedies happen and what can be done to prevent them is discussed in greater detail in Chapter 5). For this reason alone, it is essential to have a treatment plan for dealing with acute severe asthma and have the confidence to use it, knowing that it works.

As a result of their scientific training, many doctors tend to want to assess the treatments they use, and show objectively that they work. Unfortunately, the same cannot always be said for all of the alternative therapists, as we shall see in the next chapter (although, increasingly, some alternative practitioners are acknowledging that trials are needed). When it comes to acute, severe, potentially life-threatening asthma, the answer is clear; better the devil we know about than the one we don't – use orthodox medical care!

RECENT AND FUTURE DEVELOPMENTS IN ASTHMA TREATMENT

At the end of Chapter 1, I described how some doctors

are beginning to believe that inflammation is the key to asthma, a change of emphasis which has two consequences for the treatment of the disease.

Firstly, if inflammation is the main villain, then it makes sense to treat asthma primarily with anti-inflammatory drugs – such as steroids. Indeed, a number of specialists are emphasizing the need for early use of steroids in an attack: used in this way, they can often abort an attack before it gets too serious.

Advocates of this approach are not keen on the use of beta agonists, which, they say, can suppress symptoms but mask the underlying disease – which could be getting worse. Furthermore, there is a tendency for some patients given both bronchodilators and steroids to use only the bronchodilators, which have an immediate and obvious effect, and omit the steroids altogether, so doing nothing to treat the inflammation. Some specialists have even raised the possibility that over-reliance on bronchodilators could be contributing to the recent increase in the number of deaths from asthma.

Secondly, the shift in emphasis to inflammation (including the possibility that there could be persistent inflammation even in stable asthmatics) suggests that there may be other, possibly better, drugs that could be used to treat asthma. One drug which has recently appeared on the market in the UK – nedocromil – has shown promise, but the area of real excitement for many researchers lies in another group of compounds – the chemical messengers of inflammation and drugs that can block their effects. Such compounds could, at least in theory, prevent asthmatic attacks altogether – in effect, cure the disease. Routine use of such drugs is still a long way off, but who knows: not so long ago, penicillin would have been regarded as an impossibility.

3.
ALTERNATIVE TREATMENT

Alternative medicine's main contribution to asthmatics is in the field of preventing attacks. Here it is possible that it has an important role to play, particularly as the side effects of many alternative therapies are either virtually absent or notably less than those of some of the more powerful drugs used in the orthodox treatment of asthma.

As is so often the case in alternative medicine, there is unfortunately a scarcity of hard scientific evidence that these alternative therapies work. Alternative practitioners often claim that to demand such proof is to miss the point, but this is not entirely fair on patients who have a right to know whether a treatment is likely to work or not. Wise patients will also beware of the isolated glowing success story: the practitioner may have forgotten to mention the 99 patients for whom the treatment *didn't* work.

These points aside, I believe that certain alternative treatments may be genuinely helpful in asthma. Certainly, anything that can reduce the asthmatic's reliance on the more potent, potentially hazardous drugs is to be welcomed.

HERBAL MEDICINE

Herbalism is probably the oldest system of medicine there is: evidence of medical herbs have been detected in the oldest graves discovered. Even animals use herbs: for instance, cats or dogs, eating grass when they are unwell, are making use of herbs to treat themselves.

Modern herbalism is based on this very ancient tradition. Over the thousands of years that people have been trying to treat their illnesses and ailments, different herbs have been tried and experimented with. Some worked, some didn't, and as time went by, a body of knowledge was built up.

Herbals

This information has come down to us by way of the herbals written by various herbalists. These herbals are great pharmacopoeias – lists of drugs with directions for their preparation, doses and uses. The herbals evolved as they were handed down through the ages. Although the matching of herb to ailment was based on the experience of the herbalist alone, modern pharmacological methods are continually discovering that there is a scientific basis underlying many of the age-old matches.

What are medicinal herbs?

A medicinal herb is any plant that is given to a patient

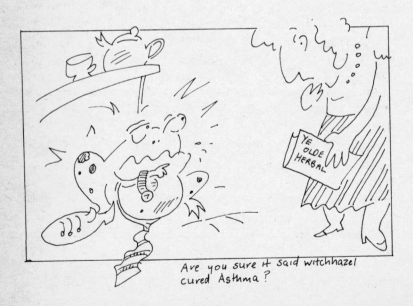

Are you sure it said witchhazel cured Asthma?

with the intention of treating their illnesses. The herbs, which are mostly used in the form of a tincture (an alcohol extract), differ from ordinary medicines in that they are derived from the whole plant, and so contain a whole host of other compounds in addition to the main compound. According to herbalists, it is these additional compounds which account for the special healing effects of herbs, as compared with the often toxic side-effects of pure drugs. Each plant is, in effect, a balanced whole medicine.

Herbs used to treat asthma

Many herbs have been used in the treatment of asthma. Those currently used include aniseed, celandine, elderflower, fennel, hyssop infusion, liquorice root, and valerian.

How herbalists treat a patient

If properly trained, a herbalist will have spent four years at a recognized college. Before starting to use herbs to treat a patient, he or she will very carefully assess the patient. The emphasis of this assessment varies between herbalists: some concentrate mostly on life-style (including diet), while others move directly to a programme of treatment based mainly on herbalism.

Some herbalists believe that life-style and diet are the true keys to the effective treatment of disease, including asthma. The herbalist will look very carefully for factors in the patient's diet which might increase the chances of the individual developing asthma. Each patient is different, and requires a separate analysis.

Once a causative factor has been identified, it is eliminated. Herbs are then used to treat any problems that remain. Other, often younger, more recently trained herbalists will approach the patient in a way more akin to those used by orthodox doctors: identifying a particular problem, and then applying an appropriate herbal remedy.

Whatever their approach, herbalists may use up to 30 different plants in one herbal medicine. More usually, however, between five and ten are used; sometimes only two or three are needed.

If a herbal treatment is going to work, it is usually apparent that it is going to do so within two weeks, and most patients can expect to be cured in six weeks. Those that don't respond probably have some other, underlying problem, and a responsible herbalist will refer the patient to a medically qualified colleague.

Throughout, however, the emphasis is on the patient as a whole, rather than on the specific symptoms. Herbs are given not so much to treat the symptoms as to heal the whole person, who will then be able to fight off the disease.

Herbalism differs from naturopathy (which has similar emphasis on life-style and diet) because of the use of herbs that is made.

Trained and recognized herbalists can be found by writing to the address given at the end of this book (page 114) and asking for a list of local practitioners.

RADIONICS

Radionics is a particularly 'fringe' therapy, and as such requires a certain amount of open-mindedness on the part of those who approach it. Bearing in mind this warning, however, it often has, according to its practitioners, a great deal to offer asthmatic patients.

In common with many alternative therapies, radionics concentrates not so much on the disease as on the individual. The emphasis is on the whole person, and the asthma and its symptoms are seen in this wider context. Even so, not all radionic practitioners use the same methods. I shall concentrate here on a fairly typical approach.

First stage in assessment

The radionic treatment starts with a comprehensive assessment of the patient, carried out by a combination of methods. The first step requires patients to fill in an

extremely comprehensive questionnaire, which covers
their family, and their past and present medical
history.

Second stage: dowsing
The second part of the assessment involves dowsing. This
is a technique that involves the use of a pendulum, which
is swung over a small sample from the patient – typically
a small length of hair stuck between two pieces of sticky
paper – known as the 'witness'. To radionic practitioners,
the witness represents the patient (this is why radionics
does not require the physical presence of the patient) and
they are able to tell, from the response of the pendulum,
the answer to their questions about the patient.

Three levels of analysis
The analysis of the patient's condition is carried out on
three levels. Firstly, there is the 'subtle anatomy', which
corresponds most closely to the concept of a patient's life
energy, or force. Next, the structures and their functional
deviation (measured on a scale of 0 to 100) are assessed:
in simpler terms, this means looking at the various
systems (such as the cardiovascular system) in the body
and determining how they are working. Finally, a cause
analysis is undertaken: this, as its name suggests,
attempts to answer the question of what may be causing
the patient's ill-health.

This very thorough analysis of the patient enables the
radionic practitioner to make a clear statement about
the patient's health. The practitioner can then proceed
to treat the patient on the basis of a comprehensive
picture of the patient.

Radionic treatment
Radionic treatment is carried out in two stages, neither
of which requires the presence of the patient. The first
step concerns 'recommendations to the patient': these
consist of suggestions as to what the patient can do to
improve his health: for example, vitamin or mineral

supplementation may be advised. Alternatively – and responsible radionic practitioners emphasize this – the practitioner may consider that radionic treatment is not suitable and that the patient therefore needs some other form of treatment (including possibly orthodox medicine), which the practitioner will recommend the patient to take up.

The second stage involves the more metaphysical elements of the treatment. Radionic practitioners believe that emanations from black boxes can be used to treat patients at a distance. They accept that this aspect of their treatment can strain the credulity of the more sceptical members of the public, but this does not bother them unduly, since as far as they are concerned, it works.

Certainly, if the claims of radionic practitioners are anything to go by, the technique works. Overall, up to 70 per cent of patients who are accepted for treatment (some patients, remember, will be advised to take other treatments) might be expected to improve to a greater or lesser extent, and of those who benefit, 20 per cent or so will show marked improvement. Only 30 per cent will show little improvement. Even when they can't cure a patient, a radionic practitioner can often say what the problem is and what treatment is likely to help.

Radionic treatment is not expensive: typical prices at the time of publication are £15 for the analysis, and £10 per month for treatment. Fully qualified practitioners, who have undergone three years training, can be contacted via the Radionic Association, whose address is given at the back of this book, on page 115.

HYPNOTHERAPY

Hypnosis, more correctly called hypnotherapy when it is used to treat disease, has had a long but chequered history. Even so, it is one of the few alternative therapies that have been relatively well accepted by the orthodox medical world. This may be because it does not require acceptance of an alternative, non-medical philosophy of health and disease before it can be used. Conventional doctors can use hypnotherapy without feeling they are undermining their traditional medical training.

No definite answer has yet been found to the question: what exactly is the hypnotic trance? It appears that it is a state of mind somewhere between sleep and wakefulness, in which subjects are able to do things they would not be able to do if they were not in a trance. While sinister uses have been suggested for hypnosis, by far the greatest use is the beneficial one of treating illness. Indeed, hypnotherapy has been used in a wide range of medical conditions, of which asthma is only one.

How hypnotherapy can prevent asthmatic attacks
Hypnotherapy does not claim to cure asthma; rather, it aims to prevent attacks. The way in which it achieves this is very simple. Although asthma is definitely not a purely psychomatic disease, there is little doubt that psychological factors can play an important role in both initiating and maintaining attacks. Especially in more 'panicky' asthmatics (as one medical hypnotherapist puts it), the fear of an asthmatic attack can provoke over-breathing, or hyperventilation as doctors call it. This greatly reduces the efficiency of breathing, and an unpleasant chain reaction is set in motion.

Hypnotherapy works by interfering with the progression to an asthmatic attack. The hypnotherapist, by inducing a state of calm relaxation, lowers the individual's tension level, so defusing the panic stage of the reaction and preventing the attack.

Initially, of course, the patient has to be hypnotized by the hypnotherapist. Once this has been done, however, the patient is taught how to put themselves into a trance – a technqiue called auto-hypnosis. Once this has been achieved, the patient uses the technique every day, typically for about 15–20 minutes, as a preventative measure. Hypnotherapists emphasize that hypnosis is not a way of treating acute attacks: these need conventional drug-based therapy. Instead, the emphasis is on preventing the attacks from developing in the first place.

As is also to be expected, hypnotherapy is of greatest help in treating patients with year-round non-allergic asthma. Panic plays less of a part in the build-up to an allergic asthmatic attack and, not surprisingly, hypnotherapy is less effective in this situation.

How effective is hypnotherapy?

Because of the large number of medically qualified doctors who use hypnotherapy, a considerable amount of worthwhile research has been done on the question of whether hypnotherapy actually works in the treatment of asthma. Most of the pioneering studies were done in the 1960s and 1970s, some of which showed that up to 75 per cent of asthmatic patients either greatly or partially improved. More average figures would be between 65 and 70 per cent.

A more recent controlled trial (see Chapter 2, pages 53 to 54, for a description of controlled trials and their importance) compared relaxation exercises with hypnosis in the treatment of asthma. The hypnotherapy group showed greater improvement and needed less drugs and time in hospital than the other group, strongly suggesting that hypnosis has something of value to offer. Interestingly, many patients, although they felt better, did not show any great change in their lung performance tests. Further research into this odd finding is being carried out.

Another, even more recent study has confirmed that mild to moderate asthmatics with a high hypnotic suggestibility can benefit from hypnotherapy.

Hypnotherapy and smoking

Hypnotherapy can also help some asthmatics in other ways. Smoking is particularly harmful to asthmatics, and hypnotherapy can be helpful in trying to conquer this self-destructive habit.

The importance of qualifications

Unfortunately, enthusiasm amongst many members of the medical profession does not prevent lay practitioners with little or no real training in hypnosis from setting up shop and advertising for patients to treat. Eminent hypnotherapists advise the public to approach only medically or psychologically qualified practitioners. The British Society of Medical and Dental Hypnosis, with about 1000 members, can provide names of local members. Its address is to be found at the back of this book, on page 114.

YOGA

Yoga is a very ancient system used to allow human beings to develop their full potential. As such, it is not exclusively a healing art (you don't have to be ill to benefit from yoga) but it does contain techniques which can be used to improve one's health, should one suffer from a chronic illness, such as asthma.

The different types of yoga

Yoga is in fact divided into various 'schools' or types, and two of these are of particular interest in treating asthma. The first of these is known as hatha yoga, and is concerned primariliy with physical postures; the second is japa yoga, which can be thought of as a kind of meditational yoga. Both (indeed all) types of yoga attach great importance to breathing.

Hatha yoga

Hatha yoga consists in the main of a series of postures, or asanas, such as the well known lotus posture. Various postures are held for varying times, while breathing and mental activity are controlled. Yogis (experts in yoga) say that the different postures benefit the body in varying ways.

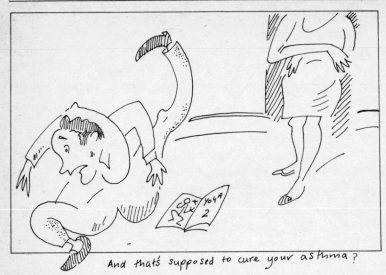

And that's supposed to cure your asthma?

Japa yoga

Japa yoga involves meditation and devotional exercises, including the mental chanting of the monosyllable 'om'. This activity, amongst other things, has been shown to calm the mind both subjectively and objectively in the laboratory.

Controlled trials

Various combinations of different yoga techniques have been tried in the treatment of asthma. More recently, there have been some controlled trials comparing yoga treatment with non-yoga treatment of asthma. Such trials have been interesting, not only for the answers they have given us about yogic treatment of asthma, but also for the broader information they have given us about controlled trials of alternative therapies in general.

One such study, recently reported in no less august a publication than the British Medical Journal, compared 53 asthmatics receiving conventional medical therapy with 53 asthmatics who followed a yogic routine, in addition to their normal therapy. The two groups had equally severe asthma, and were similar in most other respects.

·The patients' progress was followed for up to four and

a half years, although 25 dropped out during the course of the study. Statistical analysis at the end of the trial showed a highly significant improvement in the yoga group: the number of attacks per week was lowered, drug requirements were reduced and peak expiratory flow rates were improved. The authors conclude that yoga is highly beneficial in the treatment of asthma.

This study shows that it is possible to conduct reasonable scientific trials into alternative therapies. It is important to appreciate, however, that the trial only compares yoga overall with no yoga: it is not possible to say which particular element or elements of the yogic routine were responsible for the improvement. Sceptics are inclined to suggest that the benefit is due to spurious factors (like, for example, the extra attention lavished on the yoga group). Inability to refute this is one of the major problems facing trials of alternative therapies, partly because of the difficulties in devising dummy treatments which will provide the non-treated ('control') group with the same amount of attention.

The authors of the study do, however, suggest an explanation for the way in which the asthma benefits from yoga. The lungs, and in particular the airways, as we saw earlier (on page 10) are influenced by the autonomic nervous system. Other research has suggested that yoga can influence the nervous system: in particular, indicators of stress can be reduced. The authors of the study conclude the yoga may benefit asthmatic patients by reducing the amount of parasympathetic stimulation (which causes broncoconstriction) of the airways. Further studies are needed to establish whether this is the case or not.

Yoga is typical of many alternative therapies. It seems to work, but it is difficult to prove that it does, and even more difficult to say *why* it works.

HEALING

Healing, like radionics, requires a certain degree of open-mindedness to accept. Also like radionics, it requires acceptance of a system of treatment that cannot be proven by conventional scientific means. This is not to say it can't work (after all, vaccination worked before doctors understood immunology), but it does make it difficult for scientifically trained doctors to accept it. Furthermore, its underlying (and sometimes obvious) religiousness tends to put some people off.

Curing and healing: the differences

Nonetheless, healing does raise some very interesting points. Firstly, it suggests that there is more to bettering someone's health than merely curing them in the traditional scientific manner to which modern medicine has accustomed us. In fact, it actually suggests that there is a difference between *curing* an individual of a disease, and *healing* them – as a whole person.

Curing has always been focused on the disease, but this is not always what the patient wants, for it is possible to be cured without regaining full health. As the poet Matthew Prior (1664–1721) wittily put it:

> *Cur'd yesterday of my disease,*
> *I died last night of my physician*

Indeed, cures themselves are sometimes worse than the disease! Healing, on the other hand, concentrates on the patient. It is possible to be healed, without necessarily being cured.

Healers vary tremendously in their approach and philosophy. Nonetheless, there are certain themes that run fairly constantly through their work that can be identified.

Common themes in healing

One of these is the distinction between curing and healing discussed above. Another recurrent theme is the possibility that a person – regardless of what treatment they use to help another – can promote healing. Orthodox medicine recognized this phenomenon long ago, and called it the 'bedside manner'.

As a rule, healers tend to believe that they are channels through which various forces pass to their patients. If the force is believed to be strongly religious by both the healer and the patient, it may be called faith healing; otherwise, it tends to be known as spiritual healing. One thing that is virtually universal amongst healers is an inability to explain how healing actually works – beyond, that is, invoking a supernatural force or being.

This, of course, as I've already mentioned, doesn't mean that it can't work. Some healers may claim truly miraculous cures – such as cancer disappearing rapidly for no apparent reason – but the majority don't. Instead, they just state that the patient can be healed, in the broadest sense of the word.

Healing and asthma

How does all this affect asthmatics? The fact that healers vary greatly in what they claim they can achieve makes it difficult to summarize what they have to offer. The Spiritualist Association of Great Britain, for example, although they do not demand the same beliefs from their patients, consider that healing is divine intervention, and involves an intelligence far greater than that of humans. For this reason, they say, spiritual healers cannot claim to be specialists in any particular problem or promise any cures.

Other associations are more practical. There are many cases of difficult, intractable asthma which has required intensive drug therapy improving greatly after a number of healing sessions.

Comparing healing with conventional treatment

As is so often the case, the difficulty lies in proving that healing works. Answers should, however, soon be to hand (although not for asthma itself) as the Confederation of Healing Organizations are overseeing a number of clinical trials in which healing will be compared with conventional treatments. Difficult (both to understand

and to cure) diseases, such as rheumatoid arthritis, are being included in these trials, and the results, whichever way they go, will no doubt be of great interest. Certainly if healing has something to offer patients with rheumatoid arthritis, it may well have something to offer asthmatics.

If you are interested in healing, contact the Confederation of Healing Organizations at the address given at the end of this book, on page 113.

HOMOEOPATHY

Homoeopathy occupies a strange but privileged position in the world of alternative medicine. It has the seal of royal approval, of the NHS and of many doctors, and yet it is virtually impossible to prove beyond reasonable doubt whether it works, let alone *how* it works. Much of homoeopathy's success may lie, however, in its underlying philosophies.

The basis of homoeopathy

There is far more to homoeopathy than the famous principle *similaris curantur curare* ('let like cure like'). Homoeopathy was born in the days when orthodox medicine was crude, involving violent treatments, and in many ways it was a reaction against this system. The emphasis is invariably on the whole person, rather than the illness, as in the book *The Patient, not the Disease* by the famous British homoeopath Dr Margery Blackie.

Homoeopathic *treatment*, nonetheless, *is* based on the intriguing but unproven proposition that like cures like. In a series of now famous experiments at the end of the 18th century, homoeopathy's founder, Dr Samuel Hahnemann, discovered that minute doses of a particular substance could cure diseases whose symptoms were in fact the same as the symptoms produced by an overdose of that substance. Thus cinchona bark, which in overdose could produce symptoms similar to malaria, could be used in small doses to treat the disease.

Although this idea may at first sight seem a little strange, it is not completely alien to modern medicine. Immunization relies on small doses of non-virulent vaccines (harmless preparations of live or dead microbes) to provide protection against the real thing, while radiation – itself cancer-producing – is used to treat cancer.

The difficulty with homoeopathy, however, relates to the series of dilutions that are used before the substance is given to the patient. So extreme are these dilutions that it is quite possible that not one molecule of the active principle remains in the remedy that is given to the patient. Not surprisingly, the more sceptical of orthodox doctors have found it difficult to accept that these treatments could have any effect, and unfortunately, homoeopathic physicians have not to date produced definite evidence that their methods work. Nor do their explanations of *how* they work appeal to scientifically trained doctors.

Homoeopathy and asthma

Putting aside the question of scientific explanation and proof, what can the homoeopath offer the patient with asthma? First and foremost, homoeopathy concentrates on the whole person, rather than just the symptoms of the disease, for the simple reason that the same disease (and asthma is a good example) can produce different symptoms in different people.

Secondly, because many homoeopaths are fully trained conventional doctors, they are aware of and, more importantly, can recognize and treat, acute emergencies with orthodox medicines when the need arises. Thus there is little danger of a serious condition that needs urgent orthodox treatment being overlooked. Homoeopaths, for example, are unlikely to object to intensive drug-based treatment of acute severe asthma.

Homoeopathy's role in asthma is more concerned with

the day-in, day-out management of the disease. Therapy is aimed primarily at preventing attacks, rather than treating them when they have occurred. Even so, homoeopaths recognize that some asthma is allergic, and so is difficult to avoid on exposure to the causative allergen.

Homoeopathic remedies used in treating asthma
Homoeopathy, using the principle that like cures like, matches the treatment to the individual's symptoms: thus a particular remedy is indicated when the asthma mirrors the side effects of that particular substance. Inevitably, the range of potential remedies is vast, but some are used more often than others in asthma.

Arsenicum is most suited to restless patients whose asthma tends to be worse at night. Milder, emotional asthmatics are said to respond to pulsatilla. Phlegmatic asthmatics often respond to ipecac, while dry asthma responds to spongia.

Not all homoeopaths, however, agree that homeopathic treatment can be of help in asthma: indeed, one very well known homoeopathic physician said that he has 'not been greatly impressed' by homoeopathy in the treatment of asthma. Nonetheless, asthmatics who would like to find out more about homoeopathy should write to one of the addresses listed on page 114 at the end of this book.

ACUPUNCTURE

Acupuncture is one of the alternative therapies that has caught the imagination of both the lay public and the medical profession. Even the British Medical Association's report on alternative therapies, which was very dismissive of most of the alternative treatments, gave cautious acceptance to acupuncture in certain situations.

A contrast with Western medicine
What makes this all the more interesting is that the

original, authentic, Chinese method of acupuncture is based on an entirely different theory of disease to that on which Western medicine is based. Although Western scientists have tried to explain acupuncture in Western terms, no really convincing answer has emerged. We simply cannot explain acupuncture using scientific arguments, although, to be fair, there are one or two ideas that are arousing considerable interest, as we shall hear shortly.

Traditional Chinese medicine, on the other hand, has no such difficulty explaining how acupuncture works. Health and disease are explained using a totally different system to that with which we are familiar in the West.

The various organs of the body are represented in channels, called meridians, that run under the surface of the skin. Through these meridians a 'life force', or *chi* as it is known in Chinese, flows. Ill health results when there is a disturbance to the flow of *chi*, and acupuncture, by stimulating points on the meridians, corrects the flow of *chi*, so restoring good health.

Clearly, the ancient traditional system has no obvious parallel in Western medicine. Partly for this reason, and partly because acupuncture does seem to work in certain situations, attempts have been made to explain how it works using Western scientific principles. Despite some very interesting research, involving the body's own production of natural, morphine-like, pain-killing chemicals, no definite explanation has been forthcoming. As so often is the case with alternative therapies, it appears that, at least for the time being, we will have to decide *whether* it works before knowing how it works.

What an acupuncturist does

Putting aside questions about how acupuncture works, let us now turn to the question of how it is performed. As we heard earlier, disease is believed to result from disturbances in the flow of *chi* through the meridians. The acupuncturist, by selecting key points, known as 'acupuncture' points or *ah shi* points, aims to influence and so correct the flow of *chi* through the channels.

In a book of this size it is impossible to go into the details of how acupuncture points are selected. Suffice it to say that disease in one organ is often considered to be due to a malfunction in another: thus disturbances of kidney function, for example, may be related to asthma.

There are in fact several ways in which acupuncture points are stimulated, but by far the most common is through the use of needles. Fine needles, usually made of stainless steel, are inserted through the skin and directed to the *ah shi* points. In a chronic disease such as asthma, several treatment sessions may be required, with the needles being inserted for up to 30 minutes at each session.

Hazards of acupuncture

Not surprisingly for a technique which involves sticking needles into the skin, acupuncture does involve some hazards. Firstly, although it is not very painful, it is certainly not painless, and the *ah shi* points themselves can be very tender. More importantly, there are other risks. Infection is always a possibility unless the needles

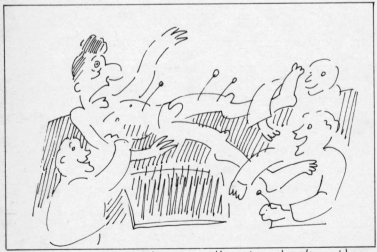

Wait – there must be an alternatwe treatment!

are kept scrupulously sterile. There is also a danger that a needle will inadvertently be placed incorrectly and damage an underlying structure. Although rare, this does happen from time to time.

But does acupuncture work in the treatment of asthma? Here again, as is so often the case, we do not have a conclusive study which will tell us one way or the other. Unfortunately, it has to be said that many of the better conducted studies have tended to suggest that acupuncture has no more than a 'placebo' effect in asthma. On the other hand, there are isolated accounts of acupuncture being of considerable benefit. Asthmatics who want to try acupuncture and decide for themselves should contact one of the addresses listed in the back of this book, on page 113.

MANIPULATION THERAPIES: OSTEOPATHY AND CHIROPRACTIC

Some chiropractors and osteopaths may not be too pleased at being considered under the same heading, but there are in fact enough similarities to justify considering the two together. Both are manipulative therapies, and, although there are differences, they have similar philosophies about the causes of diseases such as asthma.

Chiropractic

Chiropractors believe that disease is due to a misalignment, called 'subluxation', of the bones in the spinal column. The out-of-line bones press on the nerves as they leave the spinal cord, so interfering with the transmission of the nervous impulses, and in this way the disease is caused. Because nerves supply all parts of the body, it is quite possible for subluxations, through their effects on the nerves, to cause disease in any part of the body.

Osteopathy

Osteopaths explain disease in a similar way, although traditionally the disturbances are thought to be more to the blood supply than to the nerves. Although the spine is frequently implicated, it is not automatically involved, as it is in chiropractic. Osteopaths also believe that the body can be disturbed in other ways (psychologically and biochemically, for instance), and that this can cause disease. The primary defect, however, is usually structural.

Interestingly, however, when it comes to asthma, osteopaths believe that the central problem is that a disordered breathing pattern actually leads to an overstimulation of the sympathetic nervous system. More precisely, asthmatics tend to breathe using the chest muscles, rather than the diaphragm.

As some of the main nerve plexuses of the sympathetic nervous system lie in the upper chest, this pattern of breathing leads to stimulation of the sympathetic system, and before too long a vicious circle has started. Things are made even worse by the tendency to breathe through the mouth, which also leads to overstimulation of the nerve endings in the throat: this too increases the sympathetic nervous system activity.

Manipulation

Both chiropractors and osteopaths, because they consider mechanical derangement to be a major cause, if not the sole cause, of disease, use manipulation as the basis for their treatment. Chiropractors, because of the importance they attach to the spine, usually manipulate only the spine, generally using direct contact during the manipulation.

Osteopaths, on the other hand, in keeping with their broader understanding of disease, not only manipulate other parts of the body, in addition to the spine, but also use gentler techniques as well. In treating asthmatics, there are two main aims: firstly to restore abdominal (diaphragmatic) breathing, and secondly to encourage breathing through the nose. These are achieved by a combination of gentle soft-tissue (that is, non-bone) massage and gradually teaching the patient a quiet, abdominal pattern of breathing.

At no time is any undue pressure put on the patient, as stress can of course make the asthma worse. Gradually, the patient's breathing pattern should improve, and the number of attacks decrease over a period of six months or so. Osteopaths emphasize, however, that their treatment is only preventative: should an acute attack occur, the asthmatic should use medically recommended drugs to control it.

Training

Generally, osteopathic and chiropractic manipulations are carried out with great skill, and accidents are rare. All registered osteopaths and chiropractors (one should avoid unregistered practitioners) will have undergone very extensive training. Indeed, there is little doubt that, as a group, these practitioners are the most highly trained therapeutic manipulators there are: even orthodox doctors need an additional two to three years training if they are to reach the same degree of proficiency that, for example, chiropractors have.

Effectiveness

There is, therefore, little doubt about the competence of registered chiropractors and osteopaths. Furthermore, there is good evidence that in many so-called musculo-skeletal conditions (diseases affecting the muscles, bones and joints), manipulation can be very effective. The problem is establishing whether treatments such as chiropractic and osteopathy can influence diseases such as asthma which, on the face of it, have nothing to do with muscles, bones and joints.

Significantly, not all manipulators believe that their treatments should be used for all conditions, be they musculo-skeletal or not. As one leading chiropractor said, 'I think we should stick to treating the conditions we can do most for'. Certainly, this would seem to be a very sensible approach. If and when it becomes clear that manipulation benefits asthmatics (the trials have yet to be done), manipulators will be able to recommend their treatment to sufferers, confident in the belief that it will work.

Patients wishing to contact a registered practitioner should write to one of the addresses given at the back of this book, on pages 113 and 115.

SUMMARY: ALTERNATIVE TREATMENTS AND ASTHMA

Throughout this review of alternative treatments, I have emphasized the need to keep an open mind. After all, one needs scientific proof to say a treatment doesn't work just as much as one needs the proof to say it does work, and in most cases the evidence is lacking either way.

Nor is it reasonable to say that because we can't understand how a treatment works, it inevitably follows that it doesn't work. As I pointed out earlier, orthodox medicine would still be in the dark ages if it restricted itself in this way!

Complementary rather than alternative

Having said all this, we do know that, for the majority of asthmatics, and despite the side effects, most conventional treatment of asthma does work. Furthermore, when acute severe asthma threatens, orthodox treatment can be life-saving. Until we know that alternative therapies are as good as (or even better than) orthodox treatments, they should be used as *complements* rather than alternatives to conventional medicine. In this way the asthmatic can reap the benefits of both approaches, allowing the best of health with the minimum of side effects.

4.
SELF-HELP

In Chapter One we learned about the two main types of asthma – extrinsic and intrinsic. Much of this present chapter is concerned with the first type, extrinsic, or allergic, asthma: how it is caused, the mechanisms that bring it about, and, most importantly of all, what asthmatics can do to minimize their attacks. But, before we can understand how to keep attacks at bay, we need to learn something about allergy itself.

ALLERGY: WHEN THE BODY'S DEFENCES CAUSE PROBLEMS

It is only recently that doctors have started to understand allergy, and what it does. Even though they still do not know the whole story, they do believe they know enough to be able to explain the basics of allergy and the allergic response.

The immune system and how it works
Allergy has its roots in a highly specialized system we have in our bodies called the immune system. This system is something of a double-edged sword, as we shall see, but its main purpose is to defend us against infections and some other illness (certain cancers, for example, are kept at bay by the immune system: when the immune system breaks down, as it does in AIDS for example, rare cancers can develop).

The immune system works on a very simple but very elegant principle: the distinction between that which

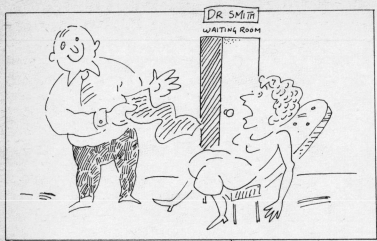

Doctor said I musn't mow the lawn, paint the house, dust the furniture, vac the carpet, and as for the barbecue tonight dear, I'm afraid you'll have to do that.

belongs to ourselves, which I shall call 'self', and that which is foreign, or 'non-self'. This is the fundamental basis of the immune system and its response, through which it identifies friend (that is, our own self) and foe, and then proceeds to attack the enemy. Let us look a little more closely at how the immune response works, taking a common childhood infection – measles – as an example.

Before we ever encounter measles, either as the disease or, more often these days, as the vaccine, we have relatively little protection against the infection. Not surprisingly, when we are exposed to someone who has the disease, we often catch it. But, unless we are very unlucky, we soon shake the disease off, and, next time we encounter it, we do not become ill: in other words, we have developed immunity to measles. How do our bodies achieve this?

How our bodies combat disease
When we catch measles, a battle is being waged within us long before we are aware that we have the disease. The virus has entered our body, and is multiplying

rapidly. At the same time, certain cells in our blood are recognizing that the virus is 'not self', and that something needs to be done about it.

These cells are the defence cells of the immune system. The first cells to be involved are known as macrophages. They recognize the virus as being non-self and ingest it (an action which in itself helps to combat the infection). The virus is then processed and presented to a second set of cells, known as lymphocytes. Once they have recognized a substance (often a protein, such as one of the proteins the measles virus is made from) they initiate the production of specific compounds, known as antibodies, which can then attack the invader. Further cells from the immune system assist by digesting the attacked measles cells, and within a few days, the measles come under control, and the patient starts to get better.

Acquiring immunity against a disease
One of the fundamental features of the immune system is that the protection doesn't end there. Once the immune system has recognized something as 'non-self', it retains a memory of the foreign object, such as the measles virus. Next time the virus is encountered, a far more rapid attack can be made, which usually manages to abort the infection before it ever gets going. When this happens, we are said to be immune to whatever the challenge is.

Two important principles of immunology can be identified from the way in which we combat measles infection. The first is that of specificity: the immune system recognizes the measles virus, and directs its attack specifically against it. Secondly, the immune system has a memory. Both of these features are of great importance in the causation of allergic asthma.

Antigens and antibodies
Before we look at asthma itself, we need to consider one aspect of the immune system in slightly greater detail. As I described above, the body reacts to the protein on

the measles virus: this protein, because it provokes the immune response, is called an antigen. In reality, not all antigens are proteins, but to be an antigen, a substance needs to possess a certain degree of chemical complexity. In nature, proteins often fit this description, which is why most antigens are proteins. It is believed that there are as many as a million antigens that can trigger an immune response in human beings.

Turning now to our own response, the chemicals that we produce to counter the antigens are also proteins, known as antibodies (also called immunoglobulins). They are divided into five classes – IgG, IgA, IgM, IgD and IgE. Of these, the last one, IgE, is the one we are most interested in, but as it is the antibody present in the smallest amounts in our blood, let us first consider the way in which antibodies behave in general.

Antibodies recognize antigens by using a 'lock and key' mechanism. Complex biological molecules have a specific shape, and antigens are no exception to this. An antibody can 'recognize' this shape, and provide a mirror image, which can then lock on to the antigen, forming a larger item known as an antigen-antibody complex.

Many antigens are, of course, hostile and disease-causing (as, for example, the measles virus protein discussed above is). Some, however, are not disease-causing in their own right, but they are capable, in susceptible people, of provoking an immune response. When this happens, and the response so triggered makes the person ill, the disease is known as an allergic disease, and the antigen that provoked the response is known as an allergen.

Extrinsic asthma: an allergic disease
Extrinsic asthma is a typical example of an allergic disease. In it, the immune system has back-fired by reacting against an allergen (antigen) which is harmless in itself. Worse still, the immune response generated actually leads to a disease – in this case, asthma.

We are now in a position to look a little more closely

at the way in which an attack of allergic asthma happens. Although many of the events in an asthmatic attack have their parallels in a healthy immune response, there are certain fundamental differences which help to explain why an asthmatic attack differs so dramatically from the more usual, beneficial type of immune response.

Atopy

Crucial to the difference is the way in which the particular cells from the immune system react to the allergen. In non-asthmatic individuals, exposure to the allergen does not lead to a response. In extrinsic asthma (and certain other diseases, as we shall see in a short while), exposure to an allergen results in over-production of a particular type of antibody – IgE. This tendency to produce excessive and inappropriate amounts of IgE is known as atopy.

Inheriting asthma

Atopy is an inherited characteristic, which is why extrinsic asthma often runs in families. Children of parents who are both atopic run a 50 per cent (1:2) chance of developing atopy, whereas the chances for an individual with no atopic relatives are only 12.5 per cent (1:8). In theory, one way in which we could help to prevent extrinsic asthma is to avoid atopic parents, but we cannot choose our parents.

Other atopic diseases

Extrinsic asthma is not the only atopic disease. In fact, the symptoms that an atopic individual experiences depend on which part of the body is most affected by the disease. Clearly in asthma it is the lungs that are affected, but in atopic dermatitis it is the skin, and in hay fever (another atopic disease) it is the nose and surrounding tissues. Not surprisingly, individuals who have one atopic disease have a tendency to develop other atopic diseases.

How extrinsic asthma occurs

Let us now return to extrinsic asthma and consider how atopy, and the excess production of IgE that it entails, causes the disease and its symptoms. To understand this, we have to bring in another set of cells, also part of the immune system, known as mast cells. Mast cells are found throughout the body (except in the brain), but it is the ones found in the lungs that concern us.

One of the most important features of mast cells is that they have large numbers of IgE receptors. A receptor is a spot on the outside of a cell which has a high affinity for a particular substance, such as a hormone or drug (or, in this case, the IgE antibody). When this substance binds onto the receptor, a response is usually triggered in the cell. A mast cell, with its large number of IgE receptors, acts like a magnet to iron filings, and binds large amounts of IgE onto its surface.

Mast cells contain quantities of various potent biological chemicals, amongst which is histamine. Histamine belongs to a class of compounds known as chemical mediators of inflammation, whose role is to act as links in the inflammatory process (as described on pages 14 to 16, inflammation is of great importance in asthma).

Mast cells also contain many other inflammation-promoting substances which have cumbersome, technical-sounding names like 'slow-reacting substance of anaphylaxis' (SRS-A), leucotriene B4 and 'platelet activating factor' (PAF). The names need not concern us overmuch – what is important is that the mast cells are potential 'bombs' containing a whole host of substances which can trigger inflammation.

Let us now return to the outside of the mast cell. Here, as I mentioned earlier, there are large numbers of IgE receptors. In atopic individuals, who have more IgE than they need, these receptors will have a high concentration of IgE attached to them. Now IgE, as we also heard earlier, is an antibody: that is, it binds to specific antigens, which in this case are allergens. As soon as any allergen enters

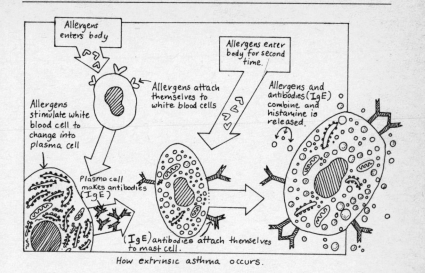

Allergens enters body

Allergens enter body for second time.

Allergens attach themselves to white blood cells

Allergens and antibodies (IgE) combine and histamine is released.

Allergens stimulate white blood cell to change into plasma cell

Plasma cell makes antibodies (IgE)

(IgE) antibodies attach themselves to mast cell.

How extrinsic asthma occurs.

the airway, it binds to the IgE concentrated on the surface of the mast cells.

Like a firing pin hitting a detonator in a shell, this is the key step. The allergen which binds to the IgE causes bridging between the IgE molecules and this in turn triggers the mast cell to undergo a process known as degranulation.

Degranulation involves the discharging of the contents of small granules contained in the mast cell into the surrounding tissues, and as it is these granules that contain the histamine and the other inflammatory mediators, inflammation results. This process acts in fact as an amplification step – small amounts of allergen can cause the release of large amounts of the inflammatory mediators.

This explains what causes the inflammation found in asthma, but what causes the smooth muscle contraction? Histamine, one of the main chemical mediators released by the mast cells on degranulation is a known stimulator of smooth muscle contraction and might seem to be a good candidate, although it does not appear to cause bronchoconstriction, at least directly. There is some evidence, however, that it might contribute indirectly, through a reflex reaction in the nervous system.

A much more likely candidate is one of the other mediators released by the mast cells on degranulation – 'slow reacting substance of anaphylaxis' (SRS-A). This substance is known to be a potent bronchoconstrictor, and although the matter is not proved beyond doubt, it is believed to be the main mediator of the bronchoconstriction that occurs in asthma. Another possible candidate (also released on degranulation) is 'platelet activating factor' (PAF).

ALLERGY AND HYPER-REACTIVITY IN ASTHMA

So far we have considered only extrinsic asthma, where the emphasis is very much on allergy. Nonetheless, there are other contributing factors, even in allergic asthma, one of which is the hyper-reactivity (over-reactivity) of the asthmatic's bronchial smooth muscle itself. In intrinsic asthma, the hyper-reactivity is of crucial importance, since it is the prime defect underlying the disease. It is also important in extrinsic asthma, but to a lesser degree, since it accounts for the non-allergically triggered attacks, such as those brought on by cold air and exercise. But whatever the trigger, mast cell degranulation is usually the final common pathway leading to an asthmatic attack, in both extrinsic and intrinsic asthma.

ALLERGEN TESTING

One of the main ways in which a patient with extrinsic asthma can help themselves is by avoiding known specific allergens. However, a note of caution is needed here. It is very easy to brand a large number of substances as allergens on the slenderest of evidence. If all such possible allergens are treated as definite allergens, asthma patients may find themselves restricting their lives to a great extent, with little or no real benefit. This

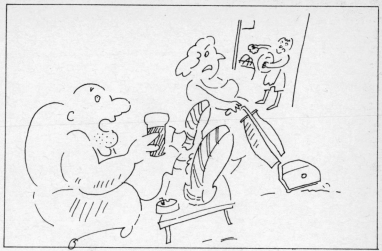

Well, it could be work I'm allergic to.

unnecessary restriction can be avoided by the use of allergy testing.

Allergy testing on the simplest level is a way of testing an individual to determine whether they are an 'allergic' person. More specific testing will determine whether an allergic person is sensitive to a particular allergen, while the most specific of tests actually assess how the lungs respond to the allergen.

Let us look first of all at the intermediate tests: those which determine whether an individual is generally allergic to a particular allergen. There are two main kinds of tests: skin tests, and the RAST (radioallergosorbent test). Both, when positive, do not prove that the allergen causes asthma, but they are of course highly suggestive. Final proof rests with a test that shows that the allergen can actually cause an asthmatic attack.

Skin tests

Skin tests, providing they are well performed, provide a straightforward and effective test. In one technique, a blob of highly concentrated extract of the allergen is placed on the skin and the skin is pricked through the a blob of highly concentrated extract of the allergen is placed on the skin and the skin is pricked through the blob. As IgE occurs throughout the body, including the skin, an individual who is sensitized to the allergen will react at the test site by producing an IgE mediated skin reaction. This reaction starts with itching and redness, and is followed by a typical weal or swelling.

Prick tests using histamine (which will definitely produce a positive result) and the extract solution without the allergen (which should produce a negative result) are done alongside the allergen test to provide standards to compare the test itself with.

RAST test

The other main test that is used to show allergy to a specific allergen is the RAST, or radioallergosorbent, test. This complicated-sounding test is in fact very simple. It is a blood test and it measures how much of the IgE antibody specific to the allergen in question is present. Serum from the patient's blood, which will contain IgE, is mixed with the suspected allergen. If the IgE antibody combines in sufficient quantity with the allergen (which it will do if the patient is sensitized to the allergen), a positive result follows. The RAST test is safer than skin testing, but it is less sensitive. It is also unfortunately more expensive, a factor of increasing importance in an ever more cost-conscious health service.

The disadvantages of RAST have resulted in skin testing usually being the primary testing method, with RAST being used as an alternative or supplementary test in selected cases.

Bronchial provocation test

Other allergy tests are sometimes used. The most specific test of all, sometimes used in situations where occupational asthma is suspected, is the bronchial provocation test. As this is a potentially hazardous test, it is performed in hospital. Increasingly concentrated solutions or, in the case of gaseous allergens, gas mixtures of the suspected allergen are inhaled until a measured effect on the airways is produced. Although in many respects this test simulates the real-life situation most closely, it does not always distinguish between allergy-induced bronchoconstriction and non-specific bronchial hyper-reactivity.

Other allergy tests

At the end of the allergy test scale are the completely non-specific blood tests for IgE and the so-called 'allergy cell' (eosinophil). Allergic individuals tend to have higher than normal levels of IgE in their blood, but the test, when positive, provides no more specific information than simply that the individual is allergic to something. Likewise the number of 'allergy cells', or eosinophils (whose true function in allergy is still something of a mystery), in the blood tend to correspond only with how 'allergic' the person is – the more eosinophils, the more allergic an individual is likely to be (though not certain to be, because other disease can cause a high count).

AVOIDANCE OF ALLERGENS

Now that we have gone through the complicated but necessary process of understanding how asthmatic attacks are triggered, we can turn to the more important practical question of what the asthmatic patient can do to minimize attacks. One of the simplest and most effective measures in the case of allergic asthma is the avoidance of allergens that cause the attacks. Sometimes, however, this seemingly so simple treatment is easier said than done. Let us look a little more closely at typical allergens, and see what can be done to avoid them.

House dust

One of the most common and widespread allergens, which unfortunately many patients with allergic asthma react to, is house dust. Research has shown that it is not house dust in general, but a specific substance in it: the faeces of house dust mites, *Dermatophagoides pteronyssimus*.

These microscopic creatures live mainly in bedding,

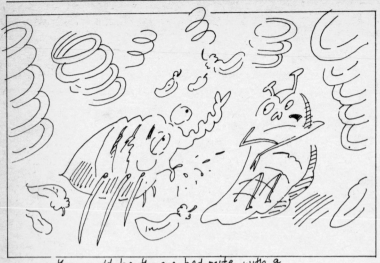

You would be the one bed mite with a feather allergy.

where they feed on a rather unsavoury diet of dead skin scales shed from our bodies. Given the right conditions, there can be over 1800 mites per gram of dust collected from our beds. Their numbers follow seasonal variations, being greatest in summer, and they prefer damp to dry conditions. They are particularly fond of any bedding that contains feathers.

These living habits clearly suggest measures that will reduce the number of house dust mites where asthmatics are sensitive to this allergen. Obviously, most of these measures apply to the bedroom, where the largest numbers of mites are to be found:

- Bedrooms should be kept scrupulously clean, and all dust removed as often as possible by hoovering and damp-dusting.
- Feather-containing bedding should be avoided, and in extreme cases a plastic sheet can be placed between the sheet and the mattress.
- Use blinds in preference to curtains, and avoid carpets as floor coverings.
- Use closed storage facilities, such as cupboards, rather than open shelves which can harbour dust.

The precautions listed will greatly reduce the number of mites, and are very worthwhile in patients with asthma that has been proved to be brought on by house dust mites, with the typical night-time attacks and positive allergen test.

Allergens from pets

Another common allergen is animal dander from a cat or other pet (scales lost from the skin of the animal, similar to the scales from humans on which house dust mites feed). Here the solution is straightforward and obvious, but often unpopular – avoid animals that cause attacks.

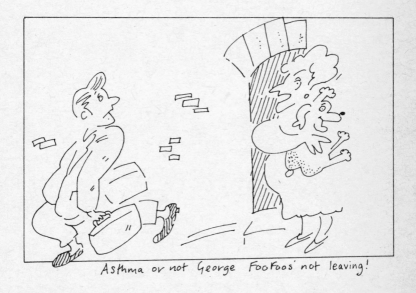

Asthma or not George Foofoos' not leaving!

Pollen

Yet another extremely common allergen is pollen. Pollen grains are actually the male sexual cell of plants, analogous to human sperm, and like sperm, pollen grains are produced in vast numbers. Luckily, however, for patients who have pollen-induced asthma, plants do not release their pollen constantly throughout the year. Nonetheless, when pollen counts are high, there is little susceptible asthmatics can do to avoid encountering the allergen, unless they are prepared to move to a pollen-free environment, such as occurs at a high altitude. Hyposensitization treatment (see page 48) can help, and is a better bet for most people.

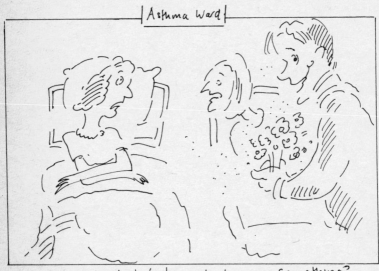

Do you think he's trying to tell you something?

Mould spores
The last group of ubiquitous allergens are the spores produced by moulds. In fact, so widespread are they that there is some difficulty in establishing whether mould spores are a specific allergen. Certainly, skin tests are often not convincingly positive, and other allergy tests are rarely of much help. If it is true that moulds cause allergic asthma, it is obviously difficult to avoid exposure altogether, although staying away from damp or decaying matter can help.

Allergies at work
Another important group of specific allergens are those classified as occupational allergens. In some cases, as with farm workers and others exposed to agricultural products, the allergen is likely to be relatively easily

identified. On the other hand, modern industrial processes, involving many complex chemicals, can make it very difficult to establish that there is a true allergy in an industrial worker. Very careful testing is necessary in these cases.

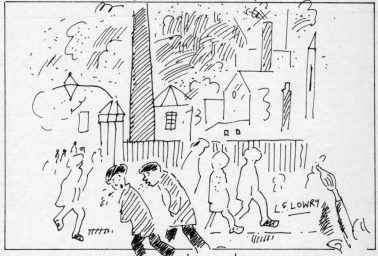

"Aye!... Ee's alreet... E' dunt' av ta breathe this stuff in all day."

Irritants

All the substances described above that can provoke asthma do so by acting as allergens through the channel of extrinsic asthma. There are, however, some substances that all asthmatics, including non-allergic asthmatics, can and often do react to. In these cases the attack is being provoked through the alternative, hyper-reactivity channel.

Most of the substances that provoke attacks in this way are moderately or very irritant, even to non-asthmatics. The difference is that the hypersensitive airways of an asthmatic react by going into bronchospasm, leading to an acute asthmatic attack. Typical substances that can cause attacks in this manner include smoke (especially tobacco smoke), sulphur dioxide (present in the air as a result of burning fossil fuels, such as coal and oil) and vapours released by new building materials. Clearly, the only way to prevent attacks caused by these materials is to avoid them.

Food allergies

Recently, and much more controversially, interest has focused on the question of whether certain foodstuffs can cause allergies that result in asthma. The most modern research suggests that up to 10 per cent of children with asthma may have some allergy to food, but even so, a direct relationship between eating the particular food and an attack of asthma is often difficult to prove. Possible allergens that could cause asthma include fish, nuts, fruits and, on rare occasions, cheese.

Food dyes and asthma

Certainly, however, there is mounting evidence that food dyes such as tartrazine can cause attacks, although it is likely that they do so through a non-allergic mechanism. Benzoic acid, used as a preservative, may also cause non-allergic asthma when eaten or drunk. Sulphur dioxide, already mentioned as an atmospheric pollutant, is used as a preservative in certain foods and drinks, such as white wine, and can provoke an attack through inhalation in susceptible people. Avoidance of known triggers will help to prevent further attacks.

Other factors triggering asthmatic attacks

Far more important are a number of very general triggers of asthmatic attacks. Exercise is a well known example, so much so that its complete absence as a trigger may make it necessary to reconsider whether the patient has asthma. Cold air is also a potent trigger.

Both of these act through the non-allergic, bronchial hyper-reactivity channel, and in fact there is good evidence that exercise-induced asthma is due not so much to the exercise itself as to the cooling effect caused by the hard breathing that exercise entails. Not surprisingly, therefore, sports which require sudden, vigorous breathing, such as sprinting, are tolerated least well by asthmatics. Long-distance swimming, on the other hand, rarely presents a problem.

Asthma and stress

One of the less well-understood possible causes of asthma is stress. In the past, beliefs have ranged from the conviction that asthma was a totally psychosomatic disease, to absolute denial of this possibility. Today, we are only marginally closer to the truth.

Certainly, most practising doctors would agree that stress and emotion seem to play a part in causing asthma. The trouble is that it has been very difficult to prove this; nor is there any obvious mechanism by which stress could cause asthma. One thing there is no doubt about is that all those who attend asthmatics – be they relatives, friends or doctors – should try to induce an air of calm whenever an asthmatic patient is unwell.

Asthmatics themselves often believe stressful situations can either cause or aggravate attacks, and in these circumstances, avoidance of difficult situations will not do any harm. Looking at the matter the other way round, an asthmatic attack can cause great anxiety for asthmatics and those attending them, which in itself cannot be helpful.

Drugs that cause asthma

One cause of asthmatic attacks over which there is no such controversy is drugs. Just as there are drugs which cause bronchodilation, so there are drugs which can cause bronchoconstriction – and thus lead to an asthmatic attack. As we heard earlier, on pages 30 to 32, beta agonist drugs are very effective in treating asthma. Not at all surprisingly, drugs which block beta receptors, such as propranolol, can aggravate asthma. These drugs, which as a group are known as beta blockers, are widely used to treat heart disease and high blood pressure, along with many other less common diseases.

Careful doctors will always check with a patient

whether they have asthma before prescribing beta blocker drugs, but as a fail-safe, asthmatic patients should always remind the doctor as well.

Another well-known drug which can cause asthma is aspirin. This common drug does not appear to cause attacks in all asthmatics, but when it does, it does so through an unusual and interesting mechanism. I described earlier how the mast cells produce the various chemical mediators that are involved in asthma, and how SRS-A is one of the more important mediators. Aspirin increases the production of SRS-A, by blocking the production of other compounds produced from the same substance SRS-A is made from, and doctors believe that the increased levels of SRS-A cause the attack.

Support for this theory comes from the fact that other drugs such as the so-called non-steroidal anti-inflammatory drugs (NSAIDs for short), which act in a similar way to aspirin often provoke attacks in susceptible patients. These individuals, who perhaps number one in five of all intrinsic asthmatics, should always avoid taking these drugs.

Infections and asthmatic attacks

Infections can also trigger asthmatic attacks: all too often patients whose asthma has deteriorated to the point where they need to go to hospital will admit that they had a cough or a cold in the preceeding few days. It is, of course, easy to see how any chest infection, with its attendant inflammation and irritation of the airways, can lead to a severe attack of asthma. All asthmatics should do everything they can to avoid getting chest infections, and should see their doctor for early treatment if they are unlucky enough to catch one.

No smoking!

Lastly (and this should hardly need to be said), asthmatics should never smoke. Also, friends and relatives who smoke can and should help by cutting down the asthmatic's exposure to smoke.

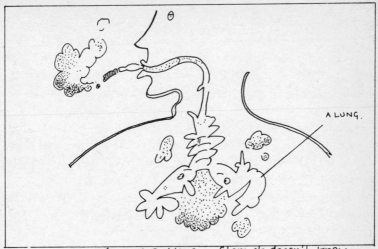

You think we've got problems — Stomach doesn't know he's going for a curry tomorrow!

ASTHMA AND AIR TRAVEL

Many asthmatics wonder whether air travel is safe for them. Generally, and certainly for mild asthmatics, there should be no problem. However, as flying in a modern passenger aircraft involves exposure to slightly lowered air pressures, and so lowered concentrations of oxygen, any patient whose asthma is sufficiently severe to cause a reduction in the amount of oxygen in the blood should take medical advice before flying.

Asthma severe enough to cause constant lowering of the oxygen in the blood is very rare, but even relatively mild chronic bronchitis can lead to reductions in the amount of blood oxygen, so a medical opinion would definitely be wise before flying. All asthmatics should of course ask to be seated in non-smoking sections of the aircraft.

ASTHMA AND PREGNANCY

In the past, asthma was seen as something of a bar to

pregnancy, but with modern knowledge and
management, this is no longer the case. Nonetheless,
asthma is the commonest lung disease that occurs in
pregnancy, and so deserves attention.

Obstetricians traditionally consider two aspects of a
medical disease occurring in pregnancy: firstly, the effect
of the pregnancy on the disease, and secondly the effect
of the disease (and of course its treatment) on the
pregnancy.

In the case of asthma, pregnancy has very little effect
on the course of the disease. Certainly, there is no
consistent evidence that pregnancy makes asthma worse,
or, for that matter, better. It is likely that the various
hormones produced in pregnancy, which have opposing
actions, tend to cancel themselves out.

Nor is there any great adverse effect of asthma on
pregnancy, either for the mother or the baby.
Occasionally, there is a tendency to slightly smaller
babies in mothers on oral steroids, or those whose asthma
is very severe, but the effect is not particularly great or
serious.

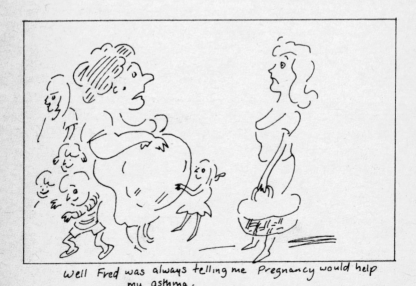

Well Fred was always telling me Pregnancy would help
my asthma.

Treating asthma in pregnancy

The treatment of asthma in pregnancy presents no great problems. Indeed, if there is any danger, it is undue reluctance on the part of doctors to use the normal anti-asthmatic drugs adequately because of the pregnancy, so exposing the mother to greater risk from the asthma! All of the usual drugs used to treat asthma (with the possible exception of steroids, as discussed below) are considered safe for both mother and baby.

Anti-asthma drugs and pregnancy

The beta agonists, such as salbutamol, have been widely used, and no problems have emerged. Interestingly, these drugs are also sometimes used by obstetricians to try and prevent premature labour, but despite this, when used to treat asthma, they do not appear to delay the onset of labour. Many obstetricians, however, do not believe that beta agonists prevent premature labour, so it may not be that surprising that beta agonists used to treat asthma appear to have no effect on the pregnancy.

Aminophylline has also been widely used in pregnancy and found to be safe. Likewise, sodium cromoglycate has never been associated with problems.

There is more controversy over the question of using oral steroids in pregnancy. Although these drugs only reach the baby in small amounts, there are concerns that they could, in theory at least, affect the baby's own steroid production. Animal experiments have also suggested that there may be an increased risk of cleft palate. In practice, however, when oral steroids have been used, none of these fears have materialized.

Nor should it ever be forgotten that asthma severe enough to need oral steroids is a serious disease, and inadequate treatment carries its own risks to the mother and her baby. Luckily, inhaled steroids do not pose the same dilemmas, as far less of the drug is absorbed into the mother's bloodstream.

Effects of pregnancy drugs on asthma

On the other hand, care is needed over some of the drugs commonly used in pregnancy. Sedatives, because they interfere with the body's breathing 'drive', should not be taken by asthmatics. Likewise, some of the drugs that can be used to induce labour can cause bronchoconstriction, and so should be avoided.

ASTHMA AND BREATHING EXERCISES

Some readers may be surprised that I have not suggested breathing exercises. This is because there is little evidence that they do any good in asthma. On the other hand, they are most unlikely to cause harm, and so need not be avoided!

5.
CHILDREN AND ASTHMA

I have devoted a whole chapter exclusively to the important subject of children and asthma for two reasons. Firstly, the problem is a frequent one: asthma is the commonest chronic chest disease of childhood – one in 10 children can expect to have asthma at some stage. It causes more lost school days than any other long-term childhood disease. Secondly, asthma in childhood can be especially frightening and traumatic – both for the sufferer, who may not understand his or her disease, and for the parents, who have to cope with the distressing sight of their chronically ill child. There is, however, much that can be done to help, as we shall see later on in this chapter.

One of the most important points to appreciate, however, is that asthma in a child is not merely adult asthma scaled down. There are additional factors that need to be taken into account, both in the disease and its treatment, as it brings with it special problems of its own.

THE NATURAL COURSE OF ASTHMA IN CHILDHOOD

Perhaps as many as one in five children wheeze at some time in their lives. Two-thirds of these children do not have true asthma, a quarter will develop intermittent asthma, while the remaining few will go on to develop severe chronic asthma. Clearly it is important to distinguish between these groups.

Most children who are going to wheeze start to do so early in life. 30 per cent begin to wheeze before their second birthday, while 80 per cent will have had their first attack by their fifth birthday. For reasons doctor's don't understand, wheezing in childhood tends to affect twice as many boys as girls. This difference between the sexes disappears during adolescence, and by adult life equal numbers of men and women are affected.

At the mildest end of the spectrum, a simple unrepeated episode of wheezing need not be called asthma. Recurrent attacks of wheezy bronchitis (viral chest infections associated with wheezing), probably *are* a mild form of asthma, and should be treated as such, although opinions do vary on this. Luckily, younger children, who are the age group who tend to get wheezy bronchitis, tend to grow out of it – 50 per cent of childhood wheezers will grow out of their condition before reaching their teens.

At the other end of the spectrum, 2 per cent or so of wheezy children will be unlucky enough to go on to develop chronic severe asthma. This is a serious disease that interferes greatly with the child's life. Growth itself can be affected, severely affected children being thinner and shorter than they might otherwise be, although they do tend to catch up with their classmates in the long run. Sometimes the child's chest takes on a characteristic barrel shape, known rather unfairly as 'pigeon chest'.

Deaths from asthma
These days, death from asthma are relatively rare. Even so, 50 or so children die tragically every year in the UK alone. While nobody wants to frighten people, it is important not to underestimate asthma's potential seriousness. Recent research has shown that asthma deaths are on the increase, especially amongst boys and young men. No explanation for this recent increase has yet been found, but it is obviously a matter of the greatest concern.

RECOGNIZING ASTHMA IN CHILDHOOD

Recognizing asthma in very young children is difficult, but as they get older it becomes easier and easier. More than three episodes of wheezing and a strong family background of allergic/atopic disease (see page 17) make the possibility of asthma very likely. Peak flow meters (see page 21) can be employed in diagnosis only if the child can use them – usually not until they are three or four. Once a peak flow meter can be used, the doctor diagnoses asthma in the same way as for an adult – by demonstrating reversible airway obstruction.

Sometimes, however, children have asthma, but do not show the classical pattern of wheezing. Such children, for example, will have recurrent coughs, which tend to be worse at night. Recognizing asthma in these cases can be difficult, as there is no wheezing to suggest what the real problem is. Unexplained recurrent attacks of breathlessness can also be due to asthma.

Three different types of childhood asthmatics
Recent research has shown that childhood asthmatics

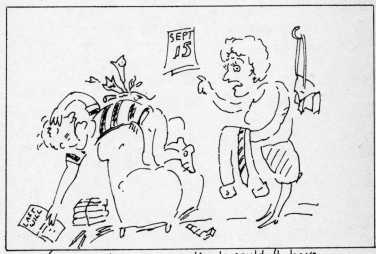

Your devastating asthma attack couldn't have something to do with it being the first day back at school?

tend to fall into one of three groups. The first group develop bouts of wheezing mainly in response to infections but in between attacks they are normal. These are the asthmatics who usually grow out of their asthma by or during their teens.

The second group have a marked tendency to develop allergic asthma. Their asthma tends to be reactive, in that it is caused by obvious external factors (which don't have to be allergens – emotionally provoked attacks also fall into this category).

The third group, which luckily contains only a few wheezy children, are the chronic severe asthmatics. Atopy is common, and the asthma, because it tends to be chronic, often leads to generalized side effects, such as the small physique and the characteristic barrel-shaped asthmatic chest ('pigeon chest') which I described earlier.

Social problems

Depending on the severity of the asthma, children suffer varying degrees of social handicap as a result of their asthma. At one end of the scale is the gregarious child who only suffers from rare, acute attacks. They are not likely to suffer any long-term ill-effects socially. At the other end of the scale are the severe chronic asthmatics who frequently miss school because of their asthma. These children are at great risk of becoming socially isolated, and every effort must be made to ensure that life is as normal as it possibly can be for them.

Chronic illness, particularly one that causes long absences from school, combined with a crippling but unobvious disability, can permanently mar an individual's social view. Extreme care is necessary to avoid the inevitable feeling of alienation that can otherwise creep in.

DIAGNOSING AND ASSESSING THE SEVERITY OF CHILDHOOD ASTHMA

As already indicated above, making a definite diagnosis

of asthma in childhood can be difficult, especially if the child is young. Nevertheless, sooner or later, one has to come down on one side of the fence and say whether the symptoms are due to asthma or not. Once this has been done, and asthma recognized, the question then becomes how to assess the severity of the disease, both overall, and at a particular moment in time.

Overall severity is assessed by taking a number of different factors into account. Doctors can learn a lot about the state of a child's asthma by asking questions and listening to the chest with a stethoscope. Likely allergens and other trigger factors can be identified, and wheezing, if present, will give a clue as to how severe the asthma is. Sometimes, however, the child is well when they see the doctor. In this situation, many doctors give the child a diary card to fill in with a record of the asthma. In this way, a picture of the asthma can be built up.

Self-assessment
Once children are old enough to use a peak flow meter – usually by the time they are three or four – assessment is made a great deal easier. These meters, or even specially developed whistles, can be used to monitor the peak flow at home as well.

Exercise tests and drug trials
Exercise tests, involving a check on how a short spell of exercise affects the peak flow, are often used, as are skin tests to confirm or eliminate the possibility of atopy. Sometimes, especially with younger patients when it is not clear whether they have asthma or not, a trial course of anti-asthmatic drugs is given. If the child improves, then it is most likely that they have asthma.

Assessing the effects on the child's life
The doctor will also want to know how the asthma is affecting the child's life: for example, how many school days are being lost because of the disease?

TREATING ASTHMA IN CHILDHOOD

Treatment of asthma in childhood has one straight-forward aim: to enable the child to live as normal a life as possible. Happily, this result is often achieved. Nevertheless, treatment is not always so successful, and for this reason it is important that certainly parents, and the children too, if they are old enough to do so, should understand their treatment so that they can achieve the best possible results.

Doctors decide what treatment to give an asthmatic child on the basis of how severe the asthma is. Clearly, patients should not be given more drugs than they need, since this will only increase the risk of side effects without achieving any benefit.

Treatment for mild asthmatics

Mild asthmatics who suffer only from isolated acute attacks, often in association with viral chest infections, do not need to take continuous therapy. Instead, they should have available a bronchodilator drug such as salbutamol, ideally taken by inhaler if the child is old

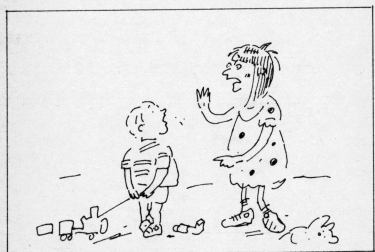

Mummy said your Asthma is psychosomatic?... but I think its all in your head

enough to manage one. This is then used, either when wheezing appears, or as a preventative measure before activities which are likely to cause an attack, such as exercise. By following such a routine, children with mild asthma can lead effectively normal lives.

Treatment for moderate asthmatics

Moderate asthma, in which attacks are fairly frequent, does require continuous therapy. More often than not, the asthma is extrinsic, so sodium cromoglycate (see page 48) is often very effective, but this drug suffers from the disadvantage that it needs to be taken three or four times a day. Alternatively, one of the slow-release aminophylline preparations can be tried, but it should be remembered that side effects are relatively more likely with this class of drugs. Whichever continuous therapy is used, children with moderate asthma should also carry a beta agonist inhaler to use whenever they feel their asthma is worsening (see page 32).

Treatment for severe chronic asthmatics

Severe chronic asthma that doesn't really respond to the above measures will usually respond to steroids. These are potent drugs, and there are additional hazards associated with their use in children, so they should only be used as a last resort. Inhaled steroids, in which the amount of drug entering the bloodstream is kept to a minimum are better than oral steroids, but sometimes, in very difficult cases, the latter have to be resorted to. In these cases, very close supervision by the doctor is necessary.

Severely affected children should also always have a beta agonist bronchodilator aerosol available to use in acute attacks. Luckily, the effects of such drugs are enhanced in patients taking steroids.

INHALED DRUGS AND YOUNG CHILDREN

One of the great problems in treating childhood asthma

is the difficulty of teaching younger children how to use an inhaler. Pressurized aerosols require considerable co-ordination, which even some adults find difficult to achieve. Not surprisingly, most children under the age of ten find it virtually impossible to master the necessary technique.

This is unfortunate, as aerosol inhalers provide a highly convenient and portable method of giving anti-asthmatic drugs. Luckily, however, there are additional and alternative devices which enable young children to enjoy the benefits of inhaled therapy.

Alternatives to standard inhalers: spacers
Part if not all of the problems with an inhaler are due to the difficulty of firing it at the right point, so that the drug goes where it is intended to go, down into the lungs. One way to get round this is to use a spacer, which also acts as a reservoir, so that the timing of firing the inhaler aerosol is less critical.

Alternatives: nebulizers
Another solution to the problem is to use a nebulizer. This device produces in effect a fine wet mist of the drug, which can easily be breathed in. Nebulizers are simple enough to be used by the youngest of children, but they suffer from the disadvantage that they require a piped supply of gas or an air compressor to drive them.

Alternatives: spinhalers
A third solution to the problem is to use a device known as a spinhaler or rotahaler. This contains the drug (often sodium cromoglycate) in a dry powdered form and releases it when the patient breathes in through the device. Children over the age of four can usually manage such a device successfully.

The failure of hyposensitization
Drug treatment of childhood asthma has shown itself to be remarkably effective and at the same time, with

modern drugs, very safe. Unfortunately, the same cannot be said for other forms of treatment such as hyposensitization. This therapeutic technique was discussed fully on pages 48 to 52; unfortunately it rarely works, even in patients with proven allergies. The poor response is believed to occur because allergy is only one of many factors involved in the causation of an asthmatic attack. Furthermore, hyposensitization also carries the risk of provoking a severe and dangerous allergic response.

ACUTE SEVERE ASTHMA

Most asthmatic children can control their asthma attacks for most of the time by following their usual treatment. Sometimes, however, their condition worsens, and the asthma responds less well to the standard measures. This is a point which all asthmatic children, or their parents if they are too young to be able to do so themselves, must be able to recognize, for it is the first and most important hint that the child may be going to develop acute severe asthma. It is the point when the asthmatic must accept that they need to see a doctor sooner rather than later.

At this point, there is no immediate urgency, as long as a doctor is seen fairly soon. While waiting for the doctor, the parents can help by keeping as calm as possible. If practical, placing the child in a hot steamy bathroom can help.

All the time, both the child and the parents should be on the lookout for signs that the attack is getting worse – once they appear, treatment is urgently needed. These clues are in fact some of the ones that a doctor uses to assess the severity of an attack, but they are equally easily recognizable by the patient and his relatives.

Signs of an acute severe attack
One of the most telling signs is being too breathless to be able to talk. Likewise, sitting forward and using the so-called accessory muscles of respiration (most obviously

seen in the neck) suggest the attack is a bad one. Turning blue is a very serious sign and indicates that *immediate* treatment is needed.

The appearance of any of these signs means that the asthmatic must be seen by a doctor, preferably in hospital as soon as possible. To delay could put the patient's life at risk. Early recognition of severe attacks is especially important because some patients die suddenly, very soon after the attack has started.

The importance of taking an attack seriously
Indeed, there is some evidence that the fatalities that do occur in asthma happen partly as a result of the asthmatic (or the parents in the case of younger children) not appreciating the severity of the attack. Failing to appreciate the gravity of the situation, they persist with their usual home treatment for far too long before calling for help. By the time they do see a doctor it is too late.

Doctors can also fail to appreciate the seriousness of an attack. Especially in hospital, with the reassuring presence of full medical facilities, it is all too easy to be lulled into a false sense of security. Constant alertness to the possibility that things may be worse than they seem is needed, if avoidable deaths are to be prevented.

All this talk of asthmatic deaths may seem a little depressing, but it is necessary. Almost all asthma deaths are, at least in theory, preventable (by recognizing that things are getting worse while there is still time to do something to rescue the patient) and anything that can help to achieve this should be done. For this reason I make no apology for emphasizing the importance of asthmatics knowing when they should call for help.

In the same vein, another avoidable factor that has been identified in asthmatic deaths is failure to take the prescribed medication. This may seem extraordinary, but it does happen. Because asthma is potentially life threatening and at the same time amenable to treatment, it is all the more important for asthmatics to understand and follow their doctor's instructions.

Modern medicine cannot cure asthma yet, but it does have the means to reduce symptoms to a minimum and avoid complications. The good news is that competent medical advice, conscientiously followed, can make life virtually normal for the great majority of asthmatics, be they children or adults.

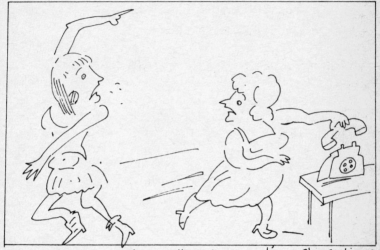

Its not an asthma attack Mum — I'm just practicing my disco dancing routine.

USEFUL ADDRESSES

Set out below, under various headings, are suggested organizations that can provide further information and/or lists of practitioners. In the case of alternative practitioners, it is important to realize that there is no legislation preventing anyone from calling themselves a therapist, even if they have no training. Where associations and registers are available, always make use of them, and only approach registered practitioners for treatment.

GENERAL

The Asthma Research Council
300 Upper Street
London N1 2XX
Tel: 01-226 2260

Asthma Society and Friends of the Asthma Research Council
St Thomas' Hospital
Lambeth Palace Road
London SE1 7EH
Tel: 01-261 0110

ACUPUNCTURE

The British Acupuncture Association and Register
34 Alderney Street
London SW1V 4EU
Tel: 01-834 1012

Can provide a register of practitioners and an
introductory handbook on acupuncture.

CHIROPRACTIC

British Chiropractic Association
5 First Avenue
Chelmsford
Essex CM1 1RX
Tel: 0245 358487

Can provide introductory leaflets on chiropractic and a
list of registered practitioners.

HEALING

National Federation of Spiritual Healers
Old Manor Farm Studio
Church Street
Sunbury on Thames
Middlesex TW16 6RG
Tel: 0932 783164

Can provide lists of healers for most parts of the
country.

HERBALISM

National Institute of Medical Herbalists
41 Hatherly Road
Winchester
Hampshire SO22 6RR
Tel: 0962 68776

Can provide leaflets on medical herbalism and lists of
registered practitioners.

HOMOEOPATHY

British Homoeopathic Association
27a Devonshire Street
London W1N 1RJ
Tel: 01-935 2163

Primarily an information service (they can provide a wide
range of publications on homoeopathy), but they also
supply a list of homoeopathic doctors.

Homoeopathic Development Foundation Ltd.
19a Cavendish Square
London W1M 9AD
Tel: 01-629 3204

Can provide a wide range of publications on
homoeopathy.

HYPNOSIS

British Society of Medical and Dental Hypnosis
Secretary: Mrs M Samuels
42 Links Road
Ashtead
Surrey KT21 2HJ
Tel: 037 22 73522

Maintains a list of medically (and dentally) qualified hypnotherapists in most parts of the country.

British Hypnotherapy Association
67 Upper Berkeley Street
London W1
Tel: 01-723 4443

Can provide leaflets and books on hypnotherapists as well as a list of practitioners.

OSTEOPATHY

General Council and Register of Osteopaths
1–4 Suffolk Street
London SW1Y 4HG
Tel: 01-839 2060

Maintains a list of registered osteopaths, who will have the letters MRO (Member of the Register of Osteopaths) after their name.

RADIONICS

The Radionics Association
16a North Bar
Banbury
Oxfordshire
OX16 0TF
Tel: 0295 3183

Supply leaflets and other publications on radionics, as well as a list of registered practitioners.

YOGA

No register of yoga practitioners exists in the same way that it does for the other therapies. Asthmatics interested in finding out more should try to find a copy of the paper in the 19th October 1985 issue of the British Medical Journal by Nagarathna and Nagendra, which describes a yogic routine used to treat asthma. Many bookshops also have introductory books on yoga that may be helpful.

GLOSSARY

Italicised words within a definition are themselves defined elsewhere in this glossary.

Accessory muscles (of respiration) – Muscles which you do not normally use to breathe with, but which can be called into play when breathing is difficult – as during an asthmatic attack.

Adrenaline – One of a variety of *hormones* produced by the *sympathetic nervous system*, which exert its effects on the body by attaching itself to an adrenergic *receptor*.

Adrenergic drugs – Drugs which mimic the effect of *adrenaline* on the body.

Allergen – A substance capable of provoking an abnormal response of the body's immune system, known as *hypersensitivity*.

Allergic asthma – Asthma in which attacks are provoked by *allergens*.

Allergy – The state in which one is abnormally sensitive to a particular substance (called the *allergen*).

Allergy testing – The process of testing for specific *allergens*.

Alpha-adrenergic agonists – Drugs capable of stimulating *alpha-adrenergic receptors* in the body.

Alpha-adrenergic receptors – One of the main types of *receptors* for *adrenergic* drugs.

Alveolar ducts – The terminal passages in the lungs that lead to the *alveoli*.

Alveoli – The minute sacs in the lungs where gases (mainly oxygen and carbon dioxide) are exchanged between the air and your blood.

Aminophylline – One of a class of drugs known as *xanthine derivatives*, used in the treatment of asthma.

Antibody – A protein produced by the body in response to an *antigen*.

Antigen – Any substance capable of stimulating an *immune response*.

Anti-histamine – A drug which blocks the effect of *histamine* on the body.

Arterial blood gases – A laboratory test used to measure the amount of oxygen and carbon dioxide in the blood.

Assisted ventilation – A form of treatment in which a patient's breathing is assisted by mechanical means.

Atopic – Having the features of *atopy*.

Atopy – A hereditary tendency to react to particular *allergens*, resulting in a number of diseases, including atopic asthma.

Autonomic nervous system – The unconscious, involuntary part of your nervous system that controls basic life processes, such as breathing and the action of the heart.

Beclomethasone – Steroid drug used in the treatment of asthma.

Beta-adrenergic receptors – One of the main types of adrenergic *receptors* for *adrenergic drugs*.

Beta-agonists (also called *beta-adrenergic agonists*) – Drugs capable of stimulating *beta-adrenergic receptors*.

Bronchial hyper-reactivity – The tendency for the *bronchi* to over-react to certain stimuli. This is one of the chief features of asthma.

Bronchial provocation test – A test used to measure *bronchial hyper-reactivity* in which lung function is measured before and after exposure to an irritant.

Bronchiole – One of the smaller airways that branch off from the *bronchi*.

Bronchitis – Inflammation of the *bronchi*.

Bronchoconstriction – Narrowing of the *bronchi* due to contraction of the muscles in their walls.

Bronchodilation – Widening of the *bronchi*, due to relaxation of the muscles in their walls.

Bronchodilator – A substance which causes *bronchodilation*.

Bronchus – Any part of the airway that lies between the trachea and the bronchioles.

Bronchi – Plural of *bronchus*.

Capillaries – The very fine blood vessels that lie between the arterial and the venous systems.

Chronic (of a disease) – Extending over a long period of time.

Chronic obstructive airways disease (COAD) – Chronic lung disease in which there is irreversible narrowing of the airways (in asthma, the narrowing is reversible).

Cilia – Very fine hairlike structures on the surface of cells that can sweep materials along by their beating action.

Clinical trial – A specific type of experiment which assesses the value of one or more forms of treatment.

COAD – See *chronic obstructive airways disease*.

Controlled clinical trial – A *clinical trial* in which one form of treatment is compared either with another treatment, or no treatment at all.

Corticosteroids – A group of drugs related to the *hormones* produced by the cortex of the adrenal gland.

Cyanosis – A blue tinge that appears on the skin, lips and nails of a patient suffering an acute attack of asthma, caused by inadequate oxygen in the blood.

Dander – Scurf, or waste skin.

Degranulation – The process whereby *mast cells* release the active compounds they contain.

Diaphragmatic breathing – Breathing using the diaphragm (the sheet of muscle separating the thorax, or 'chest' from the abdomen, or 'belly'), rather than the chest muscles, to do the work.

Eosinophilia – An increased number of eosinophils (a type of white cell) in the blood.

Emphysema – A *chronic obstructive airways disease.*

Episodic – Occuring in episodes.

Exhalation – The act of breathing out.

Expectorants – Medicines intended to make a patient cough.

Glucocorticosteroid – A particular type of *corticosteroid,* which is a powerful anti-inflammatory agent.

Histamine – A widely occurring substance in plants and animals that has a number of effects on the body.

Hormone – A substance produced in one part of the body which exerts its effects on another part, having been transported there in the bloodstream.

House dust mite – A minute insect whose faeces can provoke asthma in susceptible people.

Hydrocortisone – A specific steroid, used in the treatment of asthma.

Hyperinflation – Over-inflation of the chest due to build-up of air which is prevented from escaping by airways obstruction.

Hyper-reactivity – The tendency (of the *bronchi*) to over-react to a stimulus.

Hyposensitization – See *immunotherapy*.

Hypoxaemic – The presence of lower than normal levels of oxygen in the blood.

IgE – A particular type of *antibody* (*immunoglobulin*).

Immune response – The reaction of the body's *immune system* to foreign material.

Immune system – The system in our bodies which recognizes and counters foreign material.

Immunoglobulin – A protein that works as part of the *immune system*.

Immunology – The study of the *immune system*.

Immunotherapy – A form of treatment that aims to reduce an individual's sensitivity to a substance. Also known as *hyposensitization*.

Inflammation – The complex biological response to an unpleasant stimulus.

Inhalation – The act of breathing in.

Inhaler – A device intended to deliver a drug to a patient's lungs while they are breathing in.

Intolerance – Lack of tolerance (to a drug, such as aspirin).

Intrinsic asthma – Asthma in which *allergy* does not play a large part.

Ipratropium – A drug which causes *bronchodilation*.

Isoprenaline – A drug having actions similar to those of *adrenaline*.

Larynx – The voice-box.

Left ventricular failure – Failure of the left side of the heart (the side that pumps blood round the body).

Lymphocytes – One of many types of white blood cells.

Macrophages – Large cells which are part of the *immune system*.

Maintenance therapy – Routine treatment, aimed at keeping a disease at bay.

Mast cells – Large cells which contain granules of active substances which may be released under certain circumstances.

Mediators – The chemical messengers that bring about a biological process, for example *inflammation*.

Mucus – A sticky substance produced by various mucous membranes of the body, such as the lining of the air passages.

Nebulizer – A device which delivers a drug in the form of a mist which can be breathed in.

Oedema – The swelling of a tissue caused by the collection of excess fluid.

Parasympathetic nervous system – A division of the *autonomic nervous system*.

Paroxysmal – Occurring in attacks.

Peak expiratory flow rate (PEFR) – The maximum speed at which air can be exhaled, measured in litres per second.

Phlegm – *Mucus*, commonly known as spit, produced in the lungs.

Pigeon chest – A characteristic 'pigeon breast' shape to the chest that can arise in longstanding (*chronic*) asthma.

Placebo – A 'drug' which may make a patient feel better, but in itself has no action on the body, which can be used to eliminate psychological factors when assessing a new drug in *clinical trials*.

Prednisolone – A *steroid* drug used, along with many other drugs, to treat asthma.

Prick test – A *skin test* intended to determine the presence of *allergy* to a particular substance.

Pulsus paradoxus – A change in blood pressure that can occur in severe asthmatic attacks.

Radioallergosorbent test (RAST) – A test used to measure *allergy*, based on a measure of the amount of *antibody* in the blood.

Randomized controlled clinical trial (RCCT) – A *controlled clinical trial* in which patients are allocated at random to either the treatment or non-treatment group.

Receptor – A specialized area on or in a cell to which drugs and *hormones* become attached to bring out their effects.

Reversible obstructive airways disease (ROAD) – Lung disease characterized by reversible airways obstruction. Asthma is a typical example.

Rotahaler – See *spinhaler*.

Salbutamol – A drug which has some of the effects of *adrenaline* on the body, used to treat asthma.

Silent chest – A chest in which the asthma is so severe that hardly any air is able to enter or leave, resulting in a reduction or absence of breathing sounds.

Skin test – A test for allergy done on the skin.

Smooth muscle (also called *involuntary muscle*) – Muscle over which we have no direct conscious control.

Sodium chromoglycate – A drug believed to stabilize *mast cells*, so that they are less prone to release the substances they contain.

Spacer – A device inserted between an *inhaler* and a patient's mouth designed to increase the amount of drug reaching the lungs.

Spinhaler – A drug delivery device, which releases the drug when breathed through by the patient.

Spirograph – A laboratory machine for measuring the way in which someone breathes out.

Sputum – Dirty *mucus* and other material brought up from the lungs.

Status asthmaticus – A severe asthmatic attack which has failed to respond to normal treatment.

Steroids – A group of *hormones* and drugs that share a similar chemical make-up.

Sympathetic nervous system – A division of the *autonomic nervous system*.

Theophylline – One of a class of drugs known as *xanthine derivatives*, used to treat asthma.

Vaccine – A substance used to produce *immunity* in an individual.

Ventilation – The technical medical term for breathing.

Virus – A minute infectious parasite, that is only capable of life in a living cell.

Vitalograph – See *spirograph*.

Xanthine derivatives – A group of drugs used in the treatment of asthma.

ABOUT THE AUTHOR

CHRIS SINCLAIR, BSc, MB, BS, is both a practising doctor and a medical journalist.

A graduate of the Royal Free Hospital School of Medicine in London, he now lives in Sussex and works as a clinical assistant in Accident and Emergency Medicine at St Stephen's Hospital, London.

As a medical journalist, he currently writes for the magazines *Doctor* and *Hospital Doctor*. This is his second book.